The Heart Disease Sourcebook

The Heart Disease Sourcebook

ROGER CICALA, M.D.

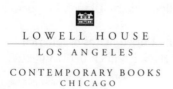

LOWELL HOUSE

LOS ANGELES

CONTEMPORARY BOOKS
CHICAGO

Library of Congress Cataloging in Publication Data
Cicala, Roger.
    The heart disease sourcebook / by Roger Cicala.
    p.   cm.
    Includes index.
    ISBN 1-56565-635-0 (cloth)
    ISBN 0-7373-0020-5 (paper)
    1. Heart—Diseases—Popular works.   I. Title.
    RC682.C556 1997   97-22199
    616.1'2—dc21   CIP

Requests for such permissions should be addressed to:
Lowell House
2020 Avenue of the Stars, Suite 300
Los Angeles, CA 90067

Published by Lowell House, a division of NTC/Contemporary Publishing Group, Inc.
4255 West Touhy Avenue, Lincolnwood, Illinois 60646-1975 U.S.A.

Text design: Kate Mueller, Electric Dragon Productions

Printed and bound in the United States of America
International Standard Book Number: 0-7373-0020-5
10 9 8 7 6 5 4 3 2

Contents

APPENDICES

Introduction

If you or someone you love has heart trouble, you are certainly not alone. Over a million Americans are diagnosed with some form of cardiovascular (heart and blood vessel) disease each year, joining 60 million other Americans who already know they have it. In the United States, over a million people are hospitalized for heart attacks every year. More than 300,000 open-heart surgeries and almost 200,000 angioplasties (nonoperative dilation of blood vessels) are performed every year.

The good news is that people with heart disease are living longer and more normal lives than ever before. New treatments and medications are more effective at keeping diseased hearts functioning and preventing heart disease from worsening. Changes in lifestyle, diet, and exercise can prevent the disease from progressing, and in some cases may actually reverse the disease process. Between 1967 and 1987, the death rate from heart disease decreased 30 percent.

In some ways, however, there has never been a worse time to be a heart disease patient. Medical research has caused confusion about which treatments are the most effective. Scandals concerning falsified research and dangerous medications have caused many people to be as afraid of their treatment as they are of the disease. At the same time, most patients find that their doctors have less and less time to explain exactly what is going on.

HMOs (health maintenance organizations), PPOs (preferred provider organizations), PROs (peer review organizations), and all the other "letter groups" have markedly changed the way medicine is practiced today. Some of these changes are for the better—more people have access to quality health care, proper medical standards are set, and costs are (at least theoretically) kept lower. On the other hand, your health-care plan may not let you go to the cardiologist or hospital you feel most comfortable with.

More importantly, almost every type of health-care plan is trying to limit expenses. This can result in fewer office visits, shortened and less frequent hospital stays, fewer tests, and denial of certain treatments and medications. At the same time doctors, who are being paid less for each procedure, are often trying to see more patients than ever. Shortened office visits mean less time for patients' questions to be answered. What could be scarier than finding out you have a potentially lethal disease and not being sure what is going to be done about it?

It's almost impossible to spend enough time with your doctor to have all your questions answered. Even when you have a lengthy discussion with your doctor, you may forget to ask some important questions until you get in the car to drive home. Hopefully, this book will fill in the question gap. This book provides a thorough discussion of what heart disease is, how it is diagnosed, what the various cardiac tests are like, and how heart disease is treated today. It also discusses the changes you can make to improve your heart's health. Finally, it includes lists of resources you can contact to find out what new information may have been discovered since this book's publication. The treatment of heart disease is changing every year, with new therapies and knowledge emerging.

A word of caution: Heart disease is not a single disease, but a group of disorders that affect the heart. Many cardiac patients have more than one type of heart disease (coronary artery disease and high blood pressure frequently occur together, for example). Others have only one type of heart disease (valvular disease, for example, is often isolated). The treatments, expectations, and tests that are appropriate for one type of heart disease may have nothing to do with another type.

If you or someone you love has heart disease, this book will help you understand what that disease is and what to expect in the future. In gaining an understanding, we can avoid the awful fear of the unknown. In some ways, that fear is worse than the disease itself.

Acknowledgments

I would like to thank Mark Heerdt, M.D., who showed me how to be a teacher, and Helen Wright, R.N., who showed me how to be a healer. And special thanks to David Dodd, M.D., as well as Cliff, Barry, Carol, and Tom, who helped me when I needed it most.

Of course, without Mom and Dad, none of this would have been possible. And most importantly, thanks to Kristin and Drew, who showed me how to be a father—the best job of all. More specifically, they usually (well, sometimes) waited their turn patiently when Dad was "playing writing on the computer."

*Nothing is less in our power than the heart,
and far from commanding we are forced to obey it.*

—Jean Jacques Rousseau

Section 1

THE TYPES OF
HEART DISEASE

Chapter 1

THE NORMAL HEART

Structure of the Heart

In order to understand the abnormalities caused by the various types of heart disease, we must have a basic understanding of the normal structure and function of the heart. The heart is not very impressive to look at, at least at first glance. It is a small muscular structure, about the size of a clenched fist, located just to the left of the center of the chest.

As seen from the outside, the lower half of the heart is made up of the large, muscular ventricles, with large veins and arteries entering and exiting from the upper half (Figure 1-1). The coronary arteries, which carry the blood supply to the heart muscle, can be seen on the surface of the ventricles.

If the heart is sliced in half lengthwise, we see that it actually contains four chambers: the left and right ventricles and the left and right atria (Figure 1-2). The walls of these chambers are made up of muscular tissue called myocardium, meaning "heart muscle." The myocardium is composed of millions of individual myocytes (muscle cells) that together form most of the heart's tissue. The myocardium is covered on the inside and outside by smooth layers of connective tissue, called the

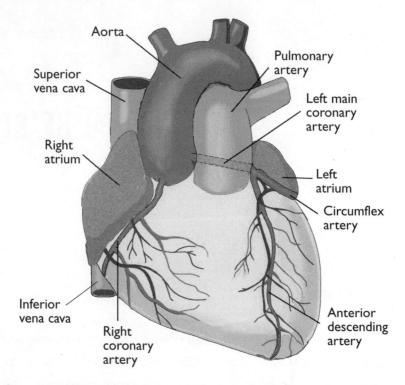

Figure I-I: *The surface of the heart as seen from the front of the body.*

endocardium on the inside of the heart and the epicardium on the out-side.

On each side of the heart the two chambers are connected in series: the small, thin-walled atrium sits above the larger, thick-walled ventricle. Blood from the veins first enters the atria and then flows into the ventricle.

Contraction of the myocytes in unison causes the chambers to squeeze into a smaller shape (just like squeezing your fist around a plastic bottle), pumping the blood out of the chamber. This contraction of the heart is called systole (SIS-toe-lee). During the period between heart contractions, called diastole (di-AS-toe-lee), the myocytes relax and the chambers get larger, allowing blood to fill both the atria and the ventricles.

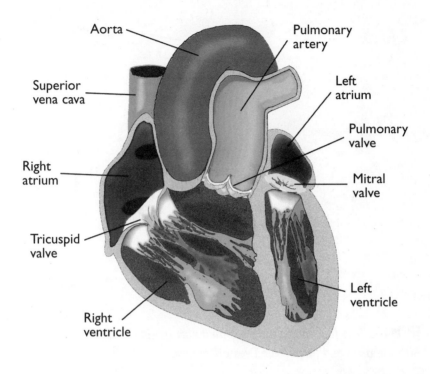

Figure I-2: *The interior of the heart.*

Between each of the chambers are valves, which are necessary to keep blood flowing in the right direction. Without the valves, contraction of the heart would pump a lot of the blood back in the direction it came from. Each valve is made up of two or three leaflets, flaps of flexible connective tissue. The valves act like one-way doors, allowing blood to flow in only one direction.

There are a total of four valves in the heart: the mitral, tricuspid, aortic, and pulmonary. The aortic and pulmonary valves are located at the exit of the right and left ventricles into the aorta and pulmonary artery, respectively. Each is made of three crescent-shaped flaps of tissue (Figure 1-3). They are sometimes referred to as the semilunar valves—their shape obviously reminded someone of a crescent moon.

The tricuspid and mitral valves are located between the atrium and

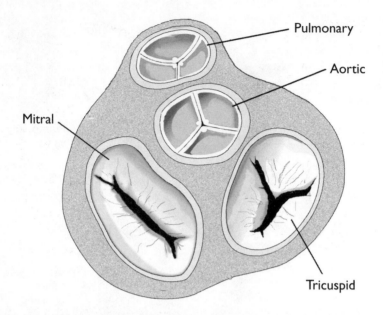

Figure 1-3: *The four major valves of the heart as seen looking from above, with the atria and major blood vessels removed.*

ventricle on the right side (tricuspid) and left side (mitral) of the heart. They are sometimes referred to as the atrioventricular valves. These valves are larger in diameter and made of thinner sheets of connective tissue than the semilunar valves (Figures 1-2 and 1-3). To keep blood from flowing backward, they are anchored to the ventricles by long threads of connective tissue, the chordae tendinae. Overall, the atrioventricular valves look a little like parachutes (Figure 1-2).

One valve is located at the entrance to and exit from each of the ventricles. During systole, when the ventricles contract, the atrioventricular valves are closed, preventing backflow of blood into the atria. During diastole, when the ventricles relax, the semilunar valves are closed, preventing blood from flowing back from the arteries into the ventricles (Figure 1-4).

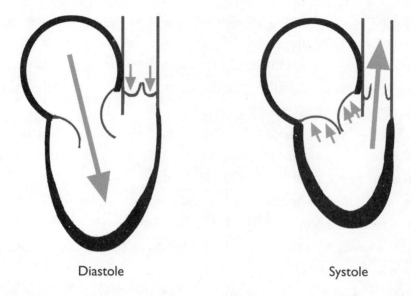

Diastole   Systole

Figure I-4: *The action of the heart valves during systole (contraction) and diastole (relaxation) of the heart.*

The Heart's Conducting System and Circulation

The heart is actually two pumps working in parallel. The right side of the heart receives blood from the body and pumps it through the lungs, where it takes up oxygen. The left side of the heart receives oxygenated blood from the lungs and pumps it out into the body.

The contraction and relaxation of the heart has to be organized in an exact rhythm. The contraction of the heart during systole consists of two phases, which correspond to the two sounds of each heartbeat. The first phase is contraction of the atria, squeezing as much blood as possible into the ventricles. The second phase is ventricular contraction, forcing blood out into the pulmonary artery (from the right side of the heart) and the aorta (from the left side).

The relaxation of the heart muscle during diastole allows the heart to fill with blood returning from the body and the lungs. Two large veins, the inferior vena cava and the superior vena cava, carry all the blood returning from the upper (superior) and lower (inferior) halves of the body and empty it into the right atrium. Several pulmonary veins bring blood from the lungs to the left atrium. Some blood also flows from the atria into the ventricles during diastole.

The rhythmic beating of the heart is controlled and coordinated by an electrical conducting system (Figure 1-5). The signal starts in a group of cells called the sinus node, located in the wall of the right atrium. These cells are the heart's natural pacemaker. Every second or so, they discharge a small electric current that travels by conducting paths to each myocyte. Several branching paths travel from the sinus node to the myocytes in the atrium, causing the atria to contract.

A second set of conducting paths transmit the electrical signal to another node of cells located near the junction of the right atrium and right ventricle, the atrioventricular node. The atrioventricular node slows the signal for about one-eighth of a second and then sends it through a large conducting system, called the His-Purkinje system, to the myocytes of the ventricles. This hesitation at the atrioventricular node allows the atria to complete their contraction before the ventricles begin to contract.

The myocytes perform a lot of work and require a large blood flow to carry the oxygen and nutrients they need. The heart itself receives about 5 percent of the blood it pumps, even though it accounts for only 1 percent of the body's weight. The blood flowing to the heart is carried through the coronary arteries, a pair of arteries that leave the aorta immediately after it exits the heart (Figure 1-1). The coronary arteries run along the outside of the heart, sending dozens of branches into the myocardium to bring blood to the myocytes.

In most people, the left coronary artery is dominant—that is, it carries the majority of the heart's blood supply. Soon after leaving the

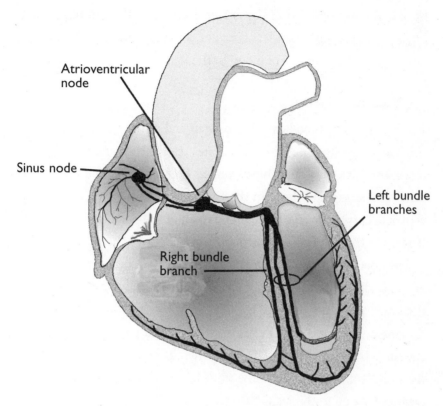

Atrioventricular node

Sinus node

Left bundle branches

Right bundle branch

Figure I-5: *The electrical conducting system of the heart.*

aorta, the left main coronary artery divides into two large branches: the left anterior descending artery and the circumflex artery. The left anterior descending artery (sometimes called the LAD) carries blood down the front of the heart, supplying both ventricles. The circumflex artery travels to the back of the heart, supplying the left ventricle. The right coronary artery, which supplies 30 to 40 percent of the heart's blood flow, also splits into two branches. The marginal artery travels along the right ventricle, supplying it with blood. The smaller posterior descending artery supplies both ventricles at the back of the heart.

A lot of variation occurs in coronary arteries. While the main branches are in pretty much the same location in everyone, they may be of different importance. For example, about 15 percent of people are "right coronary dominant." Their right coronary artery (rather than the left) carries the majority of blood to the heart.

The Circulatory System

The heart pumps blood carrying oxygen and nutrients to the tissues of the body through a network of arteries, capillaries, and veins. The arteries are thick, muscular blood vessels that carry blood away from the heart to the capillary beds in the tissues. The aorta exits from the left ventricle carrying oxygenated blood to all of the body except the lungs. It is more than an inch in diameter when it leaves the heart.

The aorta (Figure 1-1) travels upward in the chest a short distance and branches out to form the two carotid arteries, which carry blood to the brain and head, and the two axillary arteries, which carry blood to the arms. The aorta then turns back down and travels just in front of the spine through the chest and abdomen. It sends branches to the kidneys, abdominal organs, and the spine before it divides into the two iliac arteries that go to the legs.

The muscles of the smaller arteries regulate how much blood flows through them by contracting and narrowing the vessel. On a local level, this controls where blood flows. For example, when you are resting arteries to muscle tissue are contracted and only about 1 percent of blood flow goes to the muscles. When you exercise vigorously, the arteries relax and as much as 80 percent of blood flow may go to the muscles. The other effect of arterial contraction is to regulate blood pressure. If most of the small arteries are contracted, blood has to be forced forward under higher pressure.

The main arteries divide into smaller and smaller branches until they become capillaries. Capillaries are very small (only slightly wider than a red blood cell) and have extremely thin walls. As blood flows through the tissues, oxygen and nutrients pass through the thin capillary walls, while carbon dioxide and waste products from the cells flow back into the bloodstream.

The capillaries gather together to form the veins that eventually return the blood to the heart. Veins have much thinner walls than arteries because the pressure of blood in the veins is much lower. The veins from the lower half of the body come together to form the inferior vena cava, while those from the upper half empty into the superior vena cava. Both of these vessels empty into the right atrium of the heart.

The veins are much larger in diameter and more numerous than the arteries, so they can serve as a reservoir of the body's blood supply. At any given time, more than half of the blood in your body is located in the veins. At any one time, the heart, lungs, and the arteries each contain about 10 percent of the body's blood, and the capillaries about 10 percent.

Because so much blood is located in the veins, gravity sometimes can cause it to pool in the veins of the legs and abdomen when you stand too suddenly. When this occurs, very little blood flows back to the heart for a few seconds, and blood pressure falls dramatically. As a result, you may get dizzy or even faint.

As mentioned earlier, the heart is actually two pumps working in parallel. The right side of the heart receives the venous blood from the body and pumps it through the other main artery leaving the heart, the pulmonary artery (Figure 1-1), which carries deoxygenated blood from the right ventricle to the lungs. The pulmonary artery travels only a short distance before dividing into two branches that travel to the right and left lungs.

In summary, the veins bring deoxygenated blood from the body to the right side of the heart, which pumps the blood to the lungs where it receives oxygen. The left side of the heart receives oxygenated blood from the lungs and pumps it through the body (Figure 1-6).

A normal adult's heart pumps about 5 to 6 liters (a liter is about a

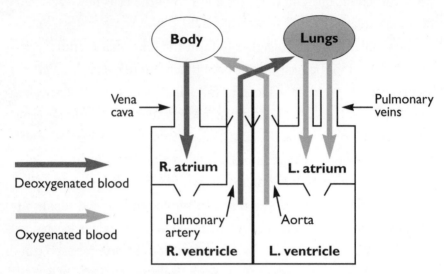

Figure I-6: *A schematic representation of blood flow through the heart.*

quart) of blood each minute. A young, healthy person's heart can pump about 24 liters a minute during vigorous exercise. At rest the heart and brain each requires about ½ liter of blood per minute, the internal organs require 3 to 3.5 liters, with the remainder of the blood flow (about 1.5 liters) going to muscle, skin, and bone. During exercise, up to 20 liters a minute goes to the muscles and a liter or more goes to the heart.

By contrast, a damaged heart has difficulty pumping more than 5 or 6 liters per minute. A person with a heart in this condition has difficulty exercising at all. A severely damaged heart may only be able to pump 3 liters of blood per minute. A person whose heart is this weakened may get short of breath just by walking a few steps.

The Different Types of Heart Disease

What we commonly refer to as heart disease or heart trouble is actually a group of diseases with different causes, symptoms, and outcomes. We classify the various types of heart disease by the part of the cardiovascular system that is most affected. By far the most common type of heart disease is hypertension (high blood pressure), which affects about 60 million Americans. Also common are coronary artery disease (narrowing of the heart's blood vessels), disturbances of the heart's rhythm, and problems with the valves of the heart.

Each type of heart disease presents its own set of symptoms. Coronary artery disease, for example, causes angina, a crushing type of chest pain that occurs when the heart does not get enough oxygen. If not treated it eventually causes a heart attack, the death of part of the heart muscle. Hypertension, on the other hand, may cause no symptoms at all.

Not surprisingly, the treatment of heart conditions is also disease specific—that is, each type of heart disease is treated with a specific set of medications or surgery. Coronary artery disease is often treated by medications that prevent the heart from working hard, minimizing the heart's oxygen needs. A completely different type of medication is used to prevent irregular heartbeats in people with rhythm disturbances.

While many people have one specific type of heart disease, many others have more than one type. This is true because the underlying conditions that affect one part of the heart are likely to affect other parts and because disease in one part of the heart stresses other parts of the heart, which may themselves fail.

An example of an underlying condition causing different types of heart disease is atherosclerosis (hardening of the arteries). Several factors contribute to the development of atherosclerosis; among them are genetic inheritance, cholesterol levels, smoking, and high blood pressure. Atherosclerosis affects arteries all over the body. If the coronary arteries are the most affected, the person may have a heart attack. If the atherosclerosis continues to progress, the person may also develop carotid artery disease leading to a stroke, or an aneurysm (swelling and weakening) of the aorta.

An example of disease in one part of the heart affecting another part is that of a person who has a heart attack caused by atherosclerosis. In a heart attack, the blood supply to a small part of the heart is totally cut off, causing heart muscle in that area to die and be replaced by scar tissue. If part of the heart's electrical conducting system is affected by the heart attack, the person may develop heart block—skipped heartbeats caused by abnormalities in the conducting system.

Certain heart conditions are more likely to exist together. For example, people with hypertension often develop coronary artery disease later in life and are also likely to develop hypertrophic cardiomyopathy (overly thick muscular walls in the heart). People with coronary artery disease are likely to develop rhythm disturbances in addition to their coronary artery disease.

Unlike the other types of heart disease, congestive heart failure almost always occurs as a secondary condition. Congestive heart failure is called the "final common pathway" of heart disease. That means that any type of heart disease that becomes severe enough, or is not treated adequately, can cause congestive heart failure. Coronary artery disease, hypertension, and valvular disease can all result in congestive heart failure if not treated effectively.

Literally, congestive heart failure is an inability of the heart to pump enough blood, resulting in congestion or backup of blood into the tissues. The symptoms of swelling, fatigue, and shortness of breath that result from congestive heart failure are what we usually think of as heart disease. Most heart patients, however, will never get to that severe stage. Even those who do can be greatly helped by new treatments and medications.

The following chapters discuss in more detail the specific types of heart disease that may affect you or your family member. Because there is so much overlap between the diseases, the treatments and diagnostic tests used for one type of disease are often used for several other types. These treatments and tests are discussed in greater detail in Section II of the book. Section III discusses the lifestyle changes that you can make to help your heart. The same changes are beneficial no matter which type of heart disease you have.

Chapter 2

CORONARY ARTERY DISEASE, ANGINA, AND HEART ATTACKS

Atherosclerosis (Hardening of the Arteries)

Atherosclerosis is a disease caused by the deposit of fat into the walls of blood vessels, especially the arteries. The disease can occur in any artery, but usually it is found in larger arteries around areas where they branch. One of the most common sites of atherosclerosis is the coronary arteries supplying the heart tissue. When atherosclerosis occurs in the coronary arteries, it is referred to as coronary artery disease.

Atherosclerosis can occur in anyone, but it is more likely to affect males, smokers, persons with high blood cholesterol levels or high blood pressure, and people who don't exercise frequently. Before age fifty, women develop atherosclerosis far less frequently than do males, because the hormone estrogen has a protective effect against the disease. After menopause, however, women are just as likely to develop atherosclerosis as men are. Those women who take supplemental estrogen after menopause retain some of the hormone's protective effects, however.

Atherosclerosis begins as small streaks of fat deposited just underneath the smooth lining of the arteries. The streaks, which usually begin near points where the arteries branch, can be found in some people as early as their late teens. As time passes, the streaks become thick accumulations of fat, known as plaques. There may be calcium deposits within the plaques, or the plaques may erode through the inner lining of the artery and project out into the lumen, the center of the vessel.

Once the plaques have become large enough to project into the artery, they may break or crack. If this occurs, the blood begins to clot over the plaque, further obstructing the artery. A piece of the eroded plaque may break off in a large artery and be carried downstream until it blocks a smaller vessel; this blockage is called an embolism. These events, the clotting or breaking up of plaques, are often the final factors that completely occlude a coronary artery, causing a heart attack.

What Causes Atherosclerosis?

Why do some people develop atherosclerosis, while others appear immune to the disease? This is not completely understood. We do know, however, of several risk factors associated with developing atherosclerosis. We cannot say for certain that an individual will or will not develop atherosclerosis, but we can say that a person is at high risk or low risk depending on the number and severity of factors present.

Some risk factors can be altered (see chapter 12), while others cannot be changed. Age, heredity, and gender are risk factors that cannot be modified. Chances of a person having atherosclerosis are directly proportional to age. Until middle age, it is much more likely to occur in men than in women. After age fifty, however, the difference between the sexes narrows considerably. Your chances of developing atherosclerosis are much higher if you have a direct family member (parent or sibling) who has atherosclerosis, especially if the relative developed it before age fifty-five.

Risk factors that can be modified include cholesterol levels, smoking, obesity, and lack of exercise. Cholesterol levels are a much-discussed factor, especially since food manufacturers have decided that low cholesterol is a marketing tool. Everyone is aware that high blood cholesterol levels are bad, but not everyone understands what cholesterol is or how it increases risk.

Cholesterol is one of the normal fats found in our bodies, where it is part of the cell membranes and various hormones. Fats don't mix with water, so cholesterol can only be transported through the bloodstream in combination with proteins that allow it to dissolve. There are two forms of this cholesterol-protein mixture: high-density lipoprotein (HDL) and low-density lipoprotein (LDL).

LDL transports cholesterol to the organs of the body, including the walls of arteries. Because LDL cholesterol is responsible for supplying the cholesterol that forms plaques, it is often called the "bad cholesterol." HDL, on the other hand, takes cholesterol from various sites in the body to the liver, where it is disposed of. HDL is the "good cholesterol," since it removes excess cholesterol from the body.

People with high levels of cholesterol, specifically LDL, are more than twice as likely to die from heart disease as are people with low cholesterol levels. (Cholesterol levels are discussed fully in chapters 12, 13, and 14; high levels are above 240 mg/dl, low levels are below 180 mg/dl.) If steps are taken to lower the cholesterol level, however, the affected person's risk drops remarkably. In fact, several studies have demonstrated that if a person achieves a 15 percent drop in blood cholesterol level (an amount that generally can be achieved by diet changes alone), the risk of heart attack is reduced by 30 percent.

Smoking is another significant risk factor that is modifiable.

Smoking reduces the amount of "good cholesterol" while increasing the amount of "bad cholesterol," thus increasing the formation of plaques. Smoking also narrows the coronary arteries and raises the pulse, increasing the amount of work the heart has to perform while at the same time reducing its blood supply. Overall, smokers are twice as likely to develop atherosclerosis and coronary artery disease as are non-smokers. The risk is tripled for heavy smokers (two packs per day). After a smoker quits, however, his or her risk drops to almost normal in about two years.

High blood pressure, itself considered a type of cardiovascular disease, is also a significant contributing factor to developing coronary artery disease. High blood pressure accelerates the development of atherosclerosis, and it also dramatically increases the workload (and oxygen needs) of the heart. When blood pressure is controlled well, the risk of both problems is reduced almost to normal.

Obesity is another risk factor for atherosclerosis for several reasons. Compared to those who are not overweight, obese people (those who weigh more than 20 percent over their ideal weight) are 50 percent more likely to have high cholesterol, twice as likely to have high blood pressure, and three times as likely to become diabetic. At the same time their heart has to work overtime to pump blood through the extra tissue created by obesity.

Other factors that increase the risk of coronary disease are diabetes (high blood sugar), lack of exercise, and a stressful lifestyle. Diabetics are much more likely than nondiabetics to develop atherosclerosis. Although diabetes may not be preventable, those who develop diabetes late in life can often minimize the severity of the disease and their risk of atherosclerosis by losing weight and eating properly.

Exercise has been shown to increase the levels of HDL while reducing levels of LDL and total cholesterol. Exercise, of course, also helps reduce weight. Over time, exercise strengthens the heart and helps it pump more efficiently. Even in a person who has already developed atherosclerosis, diet and exercise have been shown to reduce the size and severity of plaques over time.

What Are the Results of Atherosclerosis?

The plaques of atherosclerosis narrow the arteries, reducing blood flow through them. As mentioned above, pieces of plaque can also break off and flow downstream, blocking the artery where it becomes narrower and creating an embolism. Atherosclerosis can cause two other problems as well: thrombosis and aneurysm.

Thrombosis simply means the formation of a blood clot within the circulatory system. Blood usually does not clot within a blood vessel, because the interior surface of the vessel contains substances that prevent clotting. When atherosclerosis damages the vessel surface, however, these substances are no longer present. Additionally, the roughened surface of the plaque tends to signal to the clotting factors in the blood that they should become active and form a clot over the damaged area.

Such a clot can form very rapidly and narrows the blood vessel much more than the plaque itself has. If the clot completely obstructs the artery, then all the tissue that artery serves will become ischemic (deprived of oxygen) and may die. Pieces of the clot are even more likely to break off and form embolisms in the smaller vessels below the area of atherosclerosis than the plaque itself is. This clotting of plaques probably is the final step in most heart attacks and strokes. This is why people at high risk for heart attack or stroke often take anticoagulant medications, sometimes referred to as blood thinners.

If the atherosclerosis damages the wall of a blood vessel so much that it loses its strength, an aneurysm develops. When this occurs, the pressure in the vessel causes the weakened area to stretch, forming a saclike or balloonlike pouch. Aneurysms can occur anywhere but are most likely to occur in the part of the aorta located in the abdomen.

Coronary Artery Disease

Coronary artery disease is a common form of heart disease, affecting over 16 million Americans. Each year, as many as 1.5 million Americans suffer a heart attack, and 500,000 die from coronary disease. More than 600,000 invasive procedures are performed every year to treat persons with coronary artery disease, at a cost exceeding $100 billion dollars in the United States alone.

Coronary artery disease is simply atherosclerosis of the coronary arteries. As the atherosclerosis progresses, the plaques enlarge, causing the lumen (opening) of one or more of the coronary arteries to become smaller and smaller. As discussed in chapter 1, the heart muscle requires a lot of blood flow to deliver the oxygen and energy it needs to function properly. The coronary arteries deliver about ½ liter (a liter is about a quart) of blood a minute to the heart at all times, but can increase this to 1 liter a minute when the heart needs extra blood flow during exertion.

In most cases, the blockage occurs in the largest part of the artery, and near the locations where the artery branches. As the lumen gets smaller, it allows less and less blood to flow to the heart tissue. Eventually, the blood flow is so limited that the heart muscle cannot get enough oxygen to work properly.

In its earliest stages, coronary artery disease has little effect on the heart's blood flow. As the plaques enlarge, however, they block part of the artery's lumen, interfering with the amount of blood delivered. Coronary artery disease can exist for quite a while with no symptoms. At some point, sufficient blockage occurs (usually when the internal diameter of the artery is reduced to about 50 percent of its normal size) to cause ischemia—insufficient oxygen supply to the heart muscle.

What Is Angina?

The most common symptom of coronary artery disease is angina pectoris, chest pain caused by insufficient oxygen getting to the muscles of the heart. Angina is usually described as a tightness, pressure, or dull aching pain under the breastbone and on the left side of the chest. Often it is described as "feeling like someone's sitting on my chest." The pain may radiate from the chest to the left arm or the left side of the jaw, and occasionally to the back.

The symptoms of angina are experienced in different ways by different people, but an individual usually experiences the same symptoms every time an attack occurs. Many experience sweating, shortness of breath, chills, or nausea during an attack. Others have no symptoms but a mild chest discomfort. Angina usually resolves five to ten minutes after exertion stops.

Angina is caused when the muscle cells of the heart don't get enough blood flow to deliver oxygen and remove wastes. Some of the waste products, namely lactic acid and potassium, stimulate nerve endings in the heart to send a pain message. The process is almost identical to what occurs when someone develops a cramp in a leg muscle from running too far. Once the workload on the heart is decreased, blood flow is sufficient to allow it to return to normal, and the angina stops.

At first, angina usually occurs only during exertion, such as walking up a flight of stairs. It may also be brought on by exposure to cold, after taking drugs such as ergotamine (prescribed for migraine) or cocaine, and sometimes by emotional stress. All these things cause the heart to work harder, increasing its oxygen requirements. As the coronary artery disease progresses, angina occurs more frequently and with less exertion. Eventually it may occur even at rest.

While most people have the slow progression of symptoms described above, a few people experience the first symptoms of coronary disease when a blood clot or broken piece of plaque completely blocks a branch of the coronary artery, causing a heart attack. A few other people notice no symptoms when their heart muscle experiences ischemia. Such people may show signs of angina on an electrocardiogram (EKG or ECG), but if they are not evaluated by a doctor, they can have "painless angina" for years. Most of them will eventually have a heart attack.

When angina occurs in a regular pattern, such as only after a certain amount of exertion, it is termed stable angina. Stable angina is caused by a fixed blockage in a coronary artery that limits but does not totally stop the blood flow through the arteries. As long as the heart isn't working too hard, blood flow is sufficient. Overwork of the heart causes ischemia and angina, which go away after a period of rest.

When the pattern of angina changes in severity or frequency, it is referred to as unstable. The pattern may become one of less and less exercise being required to bring on an angina attack. The angina may sometimes occur while resting, or may take much longer to go away than it once did.

Unstable angina seems to occur when the plaque has progressed to the point that the lining of the blood vessel is no longer smooth. Changes in the pattern of the attacks may correspond to blood clots forming and dissolving over the plaque. Unstable angina may also occur if the coronary arteries have become irritated. Irritated blood vessels constrict, which further narrows the lumen of the artery, reducing blood flow.

Whatever the cause, we know that unstable angina tends to develop in people just before they suffer a heart attack. For that reason, any change in an angina pattern must be considered a warning of worsening coronary artery disease. A reevaluation of the severity of plaques may be necessary and new types of therapy started.

A final type of angina deserves mention because it is different in cause from the angina associated with atherosclerosis. Variant angina (sometimes called Prinzmetal's angina) occurs when coronary arteries without plaque have severe spasms. When spasm occurs, the lumen of the arteries is reduced so dramatically that angina can occur even with no atherosclerosis present. Variant angina tends to occur at night in severe but brief attacks, and most commonly occurs in women under the age of fifty. It must be evaluated like any other type of angina, however, to make certain it is not caused by coronary artery disease.

Diagnosis of Coronary Artery Disease

It can be difficult to determine whether chest pain is caused by angina. Whenever a person develops symptoms that could be angina, a complete medical evaluation is needed to determine whether coronary artery disease is present and, if so, how severe it is (see also chapter 7). The individual's medical history and descriptions of the pain, actions that cause the pain, and actions that make it better may raise a doctor's suspicion of coronary artery disease, but these factors are not sufficient for actual diagnosis. Likewise, physical examination and blood tests may show that the patient is at risk, but cannot actually diagnose the condition.

An electrocardiogram may or may not show changes of cardiac ischemia. An exercise electrocardiogram, a "stress test" done while a person is performing a specific amount of exercise, is more likely to demonstrate whether coronary disease is present. A particular change in the electrocardiogram during exercise can demonstrate that coronary artery disease is present. Even an exercise electrocardiogram is not 100 percent reliable in diagnosing coronary artery disease.

If a patient is suspected to have coronary disease, other tests must be performed to confirm the diagnosis and determine the severity of the disease. Nuclear medicine scans involve injecting thallium or technetium (two slightly radioactive chemicals that tend to "stick" to heart muscle and blood cells) into the bloodstream. After one of these chemicals is injected into the bloodstream, a nuclear detection camera can scan the amount of blood flowing to various areas of the heart. These nuclear medicine scans may be done in addition to, or at the same time as, a stress test. They not only demonstrate cardiac ischemia, but show what parts of the heart are affected.

None of these tests is absolutely accurate, however. As many as 20 to 30 percent of people with coronary artery disease have a normal preliminary examination and EKG. About 5 percent will have a normal stress EKG or nuclear medicine scan despite significant coronary disease. Additionally, 10 to 20 percent of people who have an abnormal exam do not have coronary disease. For this reason, when one of the above tests is abnormal, further invasive tests are done to visualize the coronary arteries—to determine with certainty whether disease is present, where it is located, and how severe it is.

The most direct examination of the coronary arteries is through angiography. Angiography is the injection of a radiopaque dye (one that blocks X rays) directly into the coronary arteries. X-ray movies show the dye flowing through the vessels. This allows the cardiologist to actually "see" the amount and location of disease in the arteries. Angiography will not only indicate whether coronary disease is present (Figure 2-1), but will also show in which arteries it is located and how severe the obstruction is. This information is needed to determine the best treatment.

Angiography requires cardiac catheterization. Cardiac catheterization is the insertion of a long flexible tube into an artery (usually in the groin), and the threading of the tube up through the aorta until it reaches the heart. The procedure is quite expensive and is not without risk; in a few cases it can cause heart attacks and other complications. Although such complications are rare, angiography is used only when there are strong indications that a person has coronary artery disease.

Treating Coronary Artery Disease

The main purpose of testing for coronary disease is to decide what treatment, if any, is indicated. The treatment for a given person depends on the severity of blockage and symptoms, as well as the person's overall health and age. Medical treatment concentrates on decreasing the heart's workload, which reduces the heart's oxygen requirements. Other medical therapy may be used to control atherosclerotic risk factors. Such therapy may involve taking drugs to lower cholesterol or control high blood pressure, as well as lifestyle changes.

When the condition is severe, treatment is required to reduce

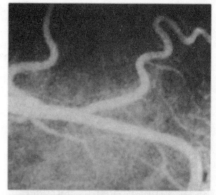
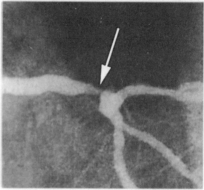

Figure 2-1: *A normal angiogram (above), and an angiogram showing 70 percent obstruction of a coronary artery (below, arrow).*

the size of the plaques that narrow the blood vessels. This may involve angioplasty, the removal or compression of plaques through a catheter inserted in the coronary artery. In other cases, a coronary artery bypass (CABG) procedure may be required. A CABG consists of removing a vein from another part of the body (usually the leg) and using it to replace (or bypass) the blocked artery.

When a heart attack occurs, treatment options depend on a host of factors. If the patient is taken to a hospital rapidly, "clot-buster" drugs may be given to attempt to dissolve a blood clot blocking the coronary artery. Alternatively, an emergency angioplasty or CABG procedure may be performed. In other cases the patient is best treated by simple supportive measures and careful monitoring while the damaged heart tissue heals.

Heart Attacks

As the atherosclerotic plaques enlarge, they become cracked and ulcerated. The clotting factors in the blood may treat this ulceration like a cut and form a clot over the plaque, completely blocking the artery. When a branch of a coronary artery becomes totally obstructed, the heart cells that it supplies die, resulting in a heart attack. Heart attack is medically referred to as a myocardial infarction, meaning death of the heart muscle.

Although clot formation over an ulcerated plaque is believed to cause the majority of heart attacks, others are caused when a piece of plaque or clot breaks off, obstructing the artery below the actual site of atherosclerosis. A few may be caused when the diseased artery contracts because of irritation from the plaque. About 1.5 million persons have a heart attack in the United States each year.

The symptoms of a heart attack are similar to angina at first, although they are usually more severe. They don't go away as time passes, however, but gradually become worse. In addition to the angina symptoms, a person having a heart attack usually feels faint or dizzy and becomes very sweaty and short of breath. Nausea and vomiting may also occur.

Whenever angina symptoms are especially severe or continue for more than fifteen minutes, the possibility of a heart attack must be considered. A few people have heart attacks that are "silent," however, causing few or no symptoms. Silent heart attacks are especially likely in elderly persons, who may note only dizziness or shortness of breath during the attack. They are also likely to occur in persons who are diabetic.

The outcome of a heart attack depends on the amount of muscle tissue destroyed and on the anatomic location of the parts of the heart affected. Outcome also depends on whether further heart attacks occur. Damage to a large amount of cardiac muscle during a heart attack can result in death from heart failure. As a general rule, damage to less than 10 percent of the heart muscle results in few long-term symptoms, while damage to more than 40 percent causes death in most cases.

If a person survives for the first two hours after a heart attack, however, chances for long-term survival are excellent. Males have a higher survival rate than do females, and persons having a first heart attack have a much higher survival rate than those having a second or third one.

Heart attack survivors may be left with some cardiac abnormalities, however. Congestive heart failure may develop, especially after second or third heart attacks. Cardiogenic shock, meaning very low blood pressure caused by severe heart failure, occurs in about 10 percent of people who suffer a heart attack. Such shock usually occurs in the first day or two after the attack and has a very high mortality rate.

If the electrical conducting system is damaged by the heart attack, dysrhythmia (abnormal heartbeats) may result. In fact, abnormal heart rhythms account for the majority of deaths that occur in the first hours after a heart attack, and half of all deaths following heart attacks. Monitoring for rhythm disturbances is the main reason patients are placed in an intensive care unit following a heart attack. Monitoring allows immediate treatment of any dangerous rhythm disturbances. Usually, the number of abnormal beats decreases markedly after the first few days following a heart attack. Permanent dysrhythmia occurs in up to half of persons who have a heart attack, but the vast majority of these abnormalities are minor and require no treatment.

Treatment of a Heart Attack

The treatment of a heart attack varies somewhat from case to case. The first rule, however, is to get the person to a hospital as soon as possible. Almost one-third of people who have a heart attack die before reaching the hospital. Of those who do get to a hospital, the vast majority will recover.

Complete cardiac arrest (meaning that the heart stops beating) can occur at any time during a heart attack. Even if cardiac arrest occurs, the patient has a good chance of survival if cardiopulmonary resuscitation (CPR) is started within four minutes of the arrest. CPR is a simple technique using mouth-to-mouth ventilation and chest compressions to pump oxygenated blood to the brain even though the victim's heart is not beating. Although CPR is a simple technique to learn, it cannot be learned from a book. CPR courses are taught by local chapters of the American Heart Association and American Red Cross. If everyone were trained in CPR, an estimated 100,000 lives would be saved each year in the United States alone.

Once a person having a heart attack reaches a hospital, medical care will proceed through several phases. In the immediate phase, emergency treatment to reduce the severity of the attack is begun. Diagnostic tests are performed to confirm that a heart attack is occurring, how severe it is, and what part of the heart is involved. If the patient is hemodynamically unstable—that is, blood pressure is not sufficient to provide blood to all the body's organs—steps will be taken to improve the function of the heart. If there are major heart rhythm disturbances, medication will be started to treat them.

Once the patient is stabilized, the care focuses on monitoring the patient for potential complications. Complications are most likely to occur within the first few days following a heart attack. If no complications occur, or when any complications have been treated and resolved, the patient begins a phase of rehabilitation along with treatment to prevent future heart attacks.

Immediate, Emergency Care

Once a heart attack has occurred, the myocytes try to protect themselves from ischemia. Whenever they are starved for oxygen, myocytes stop contracting, conserving the last of their energy. They can exist like this for up to three hours, after which time they have sustained irreversible damage and will begin to die. This three-hour period is the "window of opportunity" during which some medical treatments can actually reverse the heart attack. After this time, at least a small area of the heart muscle will have died.

The first steps taken in the emergency room are to confirm that a heart attack is occurring and, at the same time, to begin treatment. Initial treatment includes supportive measures such as administering oxygen and giving morphine for the chest pain. Morphine also dilates the blood vessels, thus reducing the workload on the heart. Nitroglycerine, another medicine to dilate blood vessels, may also be administered. In many cases, one of the beta blocker drugs is given. These drugs slow the heart's rate and decrease the force of its contraction, lowering the heart's oxygen requirements.

For the majority of patients, the initial supportive care is continued while the medical team determines how severe the heart attack is. An EKG is performed and continuous monitoring of the patient's heart rhythm is started. The final diagnosis often is made by analyzing blood to determine if it contains certain enzymes that are normally found only in heart muscle. If these are present in the blood, some heart muscle cells have died. It may take three to twelve hours for cardiac enzymes to be detected, however.

In some cases, nuclear medicine scans with thallium or technetium can also be performed to detect heart attacks. Echocardiography (ultrasound of the heart) may also be used to assess the heart's pumping action. In a few cases, emergency angiography may be performed to find the site of coronary disease, and even to treat it.

During the first hours after a heart attack (and for several days thereafter), dysrhythmias are quite likely to occur and are a common cause of death. One of the most important parts of the initial treatment, therefore, is careful monitoring to detect any dysrhythmia. As a general rule, this involves admission for several days to a coronary care unit that has continuous EKG monitoring. Medicine to treat the dysrhythmia is not given preventively, but is kept ready for use if needed.

During a heart attack, there is always some degree of heart failure, although this may be so mild that it can only be detected by sensitive tests. If the heart failure is significant enough to cause clinical symptoms, however, it must be treated medically. A large number of inotropes—medications that improve the heart's pumping ability—are available to treat heart failure. Vasodilators, which decrease the pressure that the heart must pump against, may also be used to treat heart failure. During the early period after a heart attack, these medications are usually given intravenously, since this route allows them to work almost immediately.

A patient who develops heart failure will also require invasive monitoring—catheters inserted into some of the blood vessels to measure the pressures. An arterial catheter (small tube) is often inserted in the artery at the wrist. This monitor allows measurement of the exact blood pressure generated with each heartbeat. Arterial pressure measurements allow much more accurate monitoring than a routine blood pressure taken with a cuff and stethoscope. Complications from arterial catheters are very rare.

Central venous pressure monitors (see chapter 7) are catheters inserted into the large veins under the collarbone (the subclavian vein) or in the neck (jugular vein). The catheters are threaded into the superior vena cava and right atrium of the heart, where they can measure the "filling pressure" of the heart. This allows doctors to determine the patient's fluid status. Too much fluid can worsen heart failure, while too little fluid does not allow the heart to fill properly. In about 2 percent of cases, the procedure of central venous catheter insertion causes a collapsed lung. If this occurs, another tube may be inserted into the chest to reexpand the lung.

If the heart failure is severe, it may become necessary to insert a pulmonary artery catheter. This catheter, similar in appearance to the central venous catheter, is inserted in the same place. A pulmonary artery catheter is quite long and is advanced through the right atrium and ventricle and into the pulmonary artery. This catheter allows very accurate determination of the pressures in the various parts of the heart. It can also be used to determine the cardiac output, the number of liters of blood the heart is pumping each minute. This information allows doctors to determine rapidly which medications will be of most benefit in treating the patient's heart failure.

Some heart attack patients may be treated differently, however. If a patient reaches a hospital within an hour or so after the symptoms of heart attack have begun, thrombolytic therapy may be started. Thrombolytic therapy is the use of clot-dissolving drugs in an attempt to remove the blood clot blocking the coronary artery. In thrombolytic therapy, one of several drugs may be given directly into a vein.

Thrombolytic therapy is based on the idea that heart attacks are usually caused by a blood clot forming over the plaque in a coronary artery. If the clot is dissolved, blood flow can be restored. This has to take place soon after the heart attack, before the myocytes have completely died. If thrombolytic therapy is given within two hours from the start of heart attack symptoms, almost 80 percent of patients will have restored blood flow to some degree. If it is given later than two hours, few patients will benefit.

There is currently a lot of controversy about how effective

thrombolytic therapy is and when it is most useful. Most experts agree the therapy reduces mortality if used in the first hour. Most also agree that it does not appear to be very effective for persons over seventy-five years of age, or for diabetics. The therapy does have some risks, including allergic reactions to the medication and abnormal bleeding from other parts of the body. For this reason, the treatment cannot be used in persons at risk of bleeding (ulcer patients, for example).

Angiography may be performed soon after admission for a heart attack, or it may be delayed for a few days to allow the patient to stabilize. If angiography demonstrates multiple or particularly dangerous blockages, an emergency procedure such as angioplasty may be performed to relieve the obstruction.

Angioplasty (see chapter 9) consists of inserting a small balloon at the site of the blockage during cardiac catheterization, then inflating the balloon to flatten the plaque in the coronary artery. Attempts have been made to use angioplasty, in addition to thrombolytic therapy, to relieve the obstruction during a heart attack. It is still not clear for what cases this technique is beneficial or when it should be used.

A few heart attack patients are found to have such severe, widespread coronary artery disease that emergency coronary bypass surgery is performed almost immediately. This is usually reserved for cases when it is felt that the entire left main coronary artery, or several smaller coronary arteries, are so filled with plaque that the heart attack may spread to involve these areas.

The First Forty-Eight Hours

Once a heart attack patient has been stabilized, he or she is usually transferred to a coronary care unit. Coronary care units provide constant EKG monitoring of every patient, and the personnel working in these units are skilled at diagnosing and treating the complications that are likely to develop following a heart attack. If angiography was not performed at the time of admission, it will probably be done before the patient is discharged from the coronary care unit.

Once a heart attack patient has been stabilized, the next forty-eight hours consist mostly of careful monitoring for complications. About 30 percent of patients will have further angina pain during this time and the area of heart muscle involved in the heart attack may actually enlarge slightly. If patients have had no problems or complications by the end of forty-eight or seventy-two hours, they are expected to do well and are discharged from the coronary care unit to a standard hospital bed.

Cardiac dysrhythmia is most likely to develop during this period. Almost 90 percent of heart attack patients will have premature ventricular contractions (PVCs), most of which will not require treatment. About 10 percent of patients will have ventricular tachycardia (extremely rapid heart rates from an abnormal pacemaker) or ventricular fibrillation (uncoordinated twitching of the heart with loss of the heartbeat).

Either of these latter dysrhythmias must be treated immediately with intravenous drugs. In some cases CPR or cardioversion (electric shock to restore heartbeat) may be required. Surprisingly, these dysrhythmias are more likely to occur in younger patients than in older ones. Although they are medical emergencies, the occurrence of one episode of these dysrhythmias in the post-heart-attack period does not worsen the patient's long-term outcome.

Heart failure usually develops soon after a heart attack, if it is going to occur at all. It usually becomes most severe during the first day or two after the heart attack. Obviously, patients who are in severe heart failure after the first day have a higher mortality rate than those whose heart function is near normal. If a patient remains in severe heart failure, emergency surgery or angioplasty may be attempted to help restore the heart's pumping ability.

As an alternative to surgery (or if the patient is too ill to undergo surgery), an intra-aortic balloon pump may be inserted. A balloon pump is a large mechanical device attached to a thick balloon. The balloon is inserted into the aorta through an artery in the groin. The device is keyed to the patient's electrocardiogram so that the balloon expands between heartbeats. The expanding balloon acts like a booster pump for the heart, both reducing the heart's workload and increasing its blood supply. In some cases this allows the heart time to heal and restore its own pumping ability.

Recovery After a Heart Attack

Routine Recovery

Patients who do not have complications following a heart attack can usually be discharged from the hospital in six to ten days. A few patients are discharged even sooner. Prior to discharge, patients are usually evaluated to determine the severity and extent of their coronary disease and the degree, if any, of heart failure. If coronary disease is significant, a surgical procedure or angioplasty (see chapter 9) is usually planned for the near future to reduce the risk of repeated heart attacks.

Beginning in the hospital, a cardiac rehabilitation program of gradually increasing exercise is begun. Generally, such programs take about two months to complete, but patients are expected to continue exercising on their own following the program. Patients can usually resume normal activity, such as household chores, within three to four weeks following a heart attack, although they may not return to work for six weeks to two months. Most physicians feel that sexual activity can be resumed within four weeks following a heart attack.

Part of the rehabilitation program concerns lifestyle changes to prevent worsening of the coronary atherosclerosis. Stopping smoking, reducing cholesterol intake, and improving control of high blood pressure or diabetes are important factors for reducing atherosclerosis. It has been shown that persons who make significant changes in these factors not only slow the progression of coronary artery disease, but in some cases the disease process even reverses. Such patients will actually have less coronary artery disease a year after their heart attack then they did before.

Most patients will be started on medication to help prevent future heart attacks. Mild anti-blood-clotting drugs have been shown to lessen the risk of future heart attacks in persons with coronary disease. Low doses of aspirin are commonly used, but stronger anti-clotting drugs are indicated in some people.

At the same time, medications to minimize the heart's workload are also started. Beta-blocking drugs and calcium-channel-blocking drugs (see chapter 8) reduce how hard the heart pumps and minimize the amount of oxygen the heart needs. Patients who have symptoms of congestive heart failure may need to take digitalis or another inotrope to improve the heart's pumping ability and diuretic drugs to help remove excess fluid from the body.

For many patients with coronary heart disease, surgical treatment will be recommended. The decision to recommend coronary bypass surgery or angioplasty (see chapter 9) is based on the number, location, and severity of plaques in the coronary arteries. Although both angioplasty and bypass surgery improve the condition of the majority of patients who undergo them, the procedures do have risks including further heart damage and even death. These risks are least when the procedure is performed in an institution that does hundreds of the procedures a year, and by the most experienced surgeons.

Complications

Not all heart attack patients follow the routine course of recovery. Several complications can occur during the early or late recovery periods. The vast majority of these complications are apparent by the end of the first week following a heart attack, however.

Dysrhythmia may be limited to the period immediately following a heart attack or may become chronic. In the latter case, continued medical therapy or insertion of a pacemaker may be necessary. In most cases, the dysrhythmia can be effectively treated and does not increase the patient's mortality rate.

If congestive heart failure occurs, chances of mortality after heart attack increase, in direct proportion to how severe the failure is. Patients who continue to have symptoms of heart failure despite medical therapy have a mortality rate that is much higher than that of other heart attack patients. Some forms of heart failure are caused not by loss of cardiac muscle, but by destruction of a portion of a heart valve's support structure, leading to valvular disease. In other cases of heart failure, a small section of the ventricle is so weak that it balloons out when the heart contracts, preventing much of the blood from flowing forward. These latter conditions are rare and can be corrected by surgery.

Overall, patients who survive the first week after a heart attack have a mortality rate of 6 to 10 percent during the next year. The risk of late death is higher when congestive heart failure is present, or when the patient has significant (more than 50 percent) narrowing of other coronary arteries. If there have been no further problems after one year, the mortality rate drops to 3 to 5 percent per year.

Aneurysms

Sometimes the plaques of atherosclerosis cause the wall of an artery to become so weakened that it bulges out in a balloonlike sac called an aneurysm. The most common place for an aneurysm to occur is in the aorta as it passes through the abdomen. Abdominal aortic aneurysms are more common in men than in women and usually occur in the fifties or later.

The most common symptom of an abdominal aortic aneurysm is

claudication, pain in the legs (especially the calves) when walking. The pain is caused by insufficient oxygen being delivered to the legs. Sometimes the aneurysm can cause disturbances in the gastrointestinal tract. In a few cases its first symptom is rupture and massive internal hemorrhage.

Small aneurysms may cause no symptoms and can be watched, but larger ones are likely to rupture if not removed surgically. For example, a 1.5-inch-wide aneurysm of the abdominal aorta has only a 1 in 250 chance of rupturing within a year, while a 2.5-inch-wide aneurysm has a 1 in 5 chance of rupturing during the same time. Aneurysms are also likely to develop thrombosis. Since the clot tends to remain in the ballooning portion of the aneurysm, it is a little less likely to form an embolism than are clots over atherosclerotic plaques.

Aneurysms can occur in other blood vessels, and from other causes besides atherosclerosis. Aneurysms in the blood vessels around the brain are usually not caused by atherosclerosis, but are usually the

Definitions

Arteriosclerosis: atherosclerosis involving an artery

Atherosclerosis: buildup of fatty plaques in the wall of a blood vessel, eventually causing obstruction

Cholesterol: one type of fat that is commonly involved in the atherosclerosis deposits

Coronary artery disease: disease (usually arteriosclerosis) causing obstruction of the coronary arteries

Infarction: death of tissue and cells caused by ischemia

Ischemia: insufficient blood and oxygen reaching the tissue, causing the cells to be damaged

Myocardial infarction: death of heart tissue caused by loss of blood flow, commonly called a heart attack

Plaque: a fatty deposit on an artery, found in persons with atherosclerosis

result of congenital defects in those blood vessels. They usually cause no symptoms unless high blood pressure or further weakening of the vessel from aging allows the aneurysm to rupture. Treatment of all significant aneurysms is surgical repair or replacement of the damaged blood vessel.

Kawasaki Syndrome

Kawasaki syndrome may not be a new disease, but it has only been recognized in recent years. It was first described in 1967. The disease occurs only in children, especially those under four years of age and those of Asian descent. It has replaced rheumatic fever as the most common form of acquired (rather than congenital) heart disease in children. The cause is not known, but a virus is suspected because the disease tends to occur in outbreaks, especially in the winter and spring.

Kawasaki syndrome begins as a high fever and illness that lasts from one to two weeks. There is often a rash, similar to measles, and the child's hands and feet may become red and have peeling skin. Often the eyes are also red and swollen, and the lips and tongue may become swollen and cracked. Lymph nodes in the neck are often swollen. It is important to note that these symptoms occur in many childhood illnesses; they are not specific to Kawasaki syndrome.

After one or two weeks, the symptoms of the disease improve and most children return to complete health. About one out of every four or five such children, however, develops an inflammation of the heart, especially the coronary arteries. This often results in an aneurysm and can cause coronary artery disease.

If treated, however, less than 1 percent of affected children will develop permanent heart disease. Most will return to normal health after a few months. Treatment consists of anti-inflammatory medications and immunoglobulin (human antibodies).

Chapter 3

VALVULAR HEART DISEASE

The heart contains four one-way valves (see Figures 1-2 and 1-3) that allow blood to flow only in a forward direction when the heart contracts. Valvular heart disease means that the valves have become damaged or are not functioning properly. If a valve becomes thickened or its opening is narrowed (a condition called stenosis), it is difficult for the heart to pump blood through the valve. If the valve is too weak or loose, it will allow blood to leak backward through the valve into the chamber it has just left. This backflow is referred to as regurgitation.

Many people with mild valve abnormalities have no idea they have a heart problem, and the condition is only discovered during a routine examination. Often it is discovered when a doctor listening to the heart hears an abnormal sound, called a murmur. While murmurs can occur in people with normal hearts, especially children, they may be the only sign of valvular heart disease and should be investigated.

In most cases, the heart compensates well for a damaged valve for quite a long time—often for years or decades after the damage occurs. When the valvular condition worsens, however, or if the heart weakens from other causes, the disease can cause severe symptoms and permanent damage to the heart.

Depending on the definition used, valvular heart disease is either relatively rare or one of the most common types of heart disease. Severe valvular disease that is significant enough to affect the heart's pumping ability occurs in only about 500,000 persons in the United States. Mitral valve prolapse, a mild congenital form of valvular disease, may affect as many as one of every twenty persons, however.

Structure and Function of the Heart Valves

As mentioned in chapter 1, the valves in the heart are called the mitral, tricuspid, aortic, and pulmonary (see Figures 1-3 and 1-4). The pulmonary and aortic valves (the semilunar valves) are located at the exit of the right and left ventricles, respectively. These valves have a relatively narrow opening. Because the left ventricle pumps blood at much higher pressures than the right (it pumps blood to the entire body, while the right ventricle only pumps to the lungs), the leaflets of the aortic valve are quite a bit thicker than those of the pulmonary valve.

The tricuspid and mitral valves (the atrioventricular valves) are located between the atrium and ventricle on the right and left sides of the heart. These valves have a much larger opening than the semilunar valves and are anchored to the ventricles by long threads of connective tissue called the chordae tendinae. As with the aortic valve, the mitral valve is made of thicker sheets of connective tissue and has thicker chordae tendinae than the tricuspid valve.

Problems can affect any of the heart valves, although those on the left side of the heart are more likely to have significant disease. The type of disease is generally identified by naming the affected valve along with its condition. Aortic stenosis, for example, is narrowing of the aortic valve, while mitral regurgitation is leaking of the mitral valve.

A significant amount of stenosis (narrowing) involving any of the heart valves always interferes with blood flow and must be treated. Regurgitation of the aortic and mitral valves also causes significant problems. Because the right side of the heart generates much lower pressures than the left side, regurgitation of the pulmonary and tricuspid valves is less likely to cause symptoms and rarely requires treatment.

How Valvular Disease Occurs

Valvular disease can be caused by congenital defects, by calcium deposits that form with age, or from infections of the valves. Less frequently, valves become defective because the supportive tissue around them weakens, loosening the fit of the valve leaflets. This can happen when congestive heart failure dilates the entire heart, or when an aneurysm dilates the aorta. If a heart attack weakens the heart muscle where the chordae tendinae insert, they may break, and mitral or tricuspid regurgitation can occur.

Congenital Valve Disease

Congenital valve defects occur when parts of the heart fail to develop properly. Defects of the heart valves often occur as part of a syndrome, an entire set of abnormalities and symptoms. In most cases, the valvular abnormality is only a small part of the congenital cardiac condition, which may include holes between chambers in the heart or abnormalities of the large blood vessels.

The most common forms of congenital heart valve abnormalities are aortic and pulmonary stenosis. When the stenosis is significant, the baby will have symptoms shortly after birth and surgical repair will be necessary. Milder forms of stenosis may not become apparent until adulthood, however. Ebstein's abnormality is a rare form of congenital valve disease involving the tricuspid valve. Symptoms may not occur until late childhood, and surgical repair is usually required. Mild congenital valve problems that are not discovered until adulthood occur in a very few people.

Infection

Two types of infection can cause valvular heart disease: rheumatic fever and infectious endocarditis. Rheumatic fever is caused by certain strains of streptococcus bacteria, the bacteria that cause strep throat. At one time, rheumatic fever was a common cause of valvular disease in children. Since the widespread use of penicillin to treat strep throat, it is fairly rare in the United States today, but is still a problem in other parts of the world. The number of cases of rheumatic fever has increased lately, however. Several U.S. outbreaks were reported during the late 1980s.

Rheumatic Fever

Rheumatic fever begins two or three weeks after an untreated or inadequately treated strep infection, usually in a child between ages five and twelve. An affected child develops fever and a raised, red rash on the skin. Joint pain, a rapid heartbeat, and weakness are also common. About half of the people suffering their first episode of rheumatic fever have inflammation (irritation and swelling) of the lining of the heart (endocardium) and heart valves. The mitral valve is involved in most of these cases, with the aortic valve being involved in slightly less than half.

In many cases the inflammation subsides and no permanent damage is done. In about 25 percent of cases, some permanent damage to the valves occurs. The damage is usually mild and may go unnoticed for many years. A damaged valve tends to worsen slowly over time, however, and fifteen to thirty years after an episode of rheumatic fever, the damage may become severe enough to cause symptoms or require repair.

Infective Endocarditis

Infective endocarditis is a bacterial infection of the heart valves and endocardium. Because endocarditis involves an actual infection of the valve (not simple inflammation like rheumatic fever), it is usually a severe, life-threatening illness. Often weeks of intravenous antibiotics are required to remove the infection. Endocarditis can occur whenever bacteria enter the bloodstream, but it usually occurs in people who already have minor valve damage.

The infecting bacteria cause valve damage. If the infection is cleared fairly rapidly, the damage may be limited, although like all valve damage it may slowly worsen over time. Severe infection may almost totally destroy one or more heart valves, requiring emergency surgery to replace the valve with an artificial one. Doctors will try to avoid replacing a valve until the infection is completely cleared, since artificial valves serve as a site for bacteria to "hide" from the body's immune system.

Persons with minor valve problems must be extremely careful to avoid endocarditis, since they are at high risk to develop it whenever any bacteria enter their bloodstream. This includes persons with congenital heart disease, those who have had rheumatic fever, and probably those with significant mitral valve prolapse. Whenever such people have surgery of any kind (including dental surgery) or suffer any type of bacterial infection, they should be treated with preventive antibiotics.

Other Causes of Valve Disease

Valvular disease can occur from a variety of other causes. Stenosis of the valves may occur during the aging process as connective tissue thickens and becomes stiff. If the structures that support the valve become weakened, the valve loosens and may become regurgitant. This can occur if the support structure is involved in a heart attack, if the heart becomes dilated (enlarged) from congestive heart failure, or if the heart or aorta develops an aneurysm. Very rarely, a valve can be physically damaged during open-heart surgery or during insertion of a catheter into the heart for diagnostic reasons.

The Major Categories of Valve Disease

When doctors classify valvular heart disease, they generally label the problem by stating the valve involved, and whether the valve is stenotic (narrowed opening) or regurgitant (leaking). In most cases, they won't include the cause of the disease, often because the original cause is unknown, but also because the cause usually does not influence the outcome or treatment of the problem. These are determined solely by the severity of the valvular defects.

The valves on the left side of the heart—the mitral valve between the atrium and ventricle and the aortic valve between the ventricle and aorta—are more commonly involved in valvular disease and will be discussed in detail below. When valvular disease affects the right side of the heart, it is usually less significant because the pressures on the right side of the heart are much lower.

Mitral Stenosis

Mitral stenosis is most commonly caused by childhood rheumatic fever, although its symptoms may not become apparent until the affected person is a young adult. Less frequently, mitral stenosis occurs in old age, usually from calcium deposits in the valve itself. Some other cases are idiopathic, that is, the cause is unknown. Mitral stenosis is much less common today in the United States than it was thirty years ago, because rheumatic fever has been controlled. It is still very common in Third World countries, however.

In mild cases of mitral stenosis, the opening of the valve is slightly narrowed, but the heart functions normally. As the severity of mitral stenosis increases, blood backs up in the left atrium. Over time the atrium distends and its wall becomes thickened as it tries to force blood through the tight valve. As the condition worsens, pressure causes blood to back up through the pulmonary veins into the lungs. This can result in fluid collection in the lungs (pulmonary edema).

When the left atrium enlarges, it may develop rhythm irregularities and no longer contract properly. The most common rhythm irregularity is atrial fibrillation, a rapid vibrating of the atria with no true contraction. Because blood tends to pool in the atrium without moving, it may clot. If a piece of blood clot breaks off, it may flow through the heart and obstruct an artery to the brain, causing a stroke.

Mild mitral stenosis causes almost no symptoms. Many people with mild disease remain almost symptom free for decades. If the disease progresses, affected persons usually notice fatigue or shortness of breath during mild exercise. When pulmonary edema develops, they may suffer shortness of breath whenever they lie flat (this is called orthopnea) or suddenly awake short of breath in the middle of the night (this is called aroxysmal nocturnal dyspnea). Atrial fibrillation usually develops in only the most advanced cases.

Persons with mild degrees of mitral stenosis generally require only prophylactic antibiotics to prevent infective endocarditis. As the disease progresses, echocardiography may be performed to visualize the severity of the stenosis, and a cardiac catheterization may be performed to measure the pressures generated by the condition. In some cases, the valve may be stretched open using a balloon during cardiac catheterization. Severe cases will require replacement of the valve.

Mitral Regurgitation

Mitral regurgitation occurs more commonly than does mitral stenosis. It can be caused by infection of the valve's leaflets or by a heart attack that has destroyed some of the papillary muscles (see Figure 1-4) that support the leaflets. Less commonly, mitral valve prolapse can worsen to the point that the valve begins to leak.

When the mitral valve leaks, some of the blood that should flow out into the aorta instead flows back into the left atrium through the mitral valve. This decreases the amount of blood flowing out to the body with each heartbeat, lowering the blood pressure. It also increases the work of the left atrium, since it must pump this regurgitated blood back into the left ventricle for the next heartbeat.

The symptoms of mitral regurgitation vary a lot depending on whether the condition develops suddenly (such as following a heart attack) or slowly (from worsening mitral valve prolapse, for example). If the condition develops rapidly, the affected person becomes suddenly short of breath and may faint. The person often finds the symptoms are worse when lying down and will attempt to sit up.

If the condition develops slowly, the heart enlarges and compensates to a large degree, much better than it does for stenosis. Often the condition becomes quite advanced before there are many symptoms. Eventually, the affected person develops fatigue, weakness, and shortness of breath. The symptoms of pulmonary edema described above also occur, as may fluid retention and swelling in the ankles.

When mitral valve regurgitation develops suddenly, emergency surgical replacement of the valve is usually required. Chronic or slowly developing mitral valve prolapse presents a different problem. Often persons with significant mitral valve prolapse will have few symptoms and feel they can live with the condition. If the valve is not replaced, however, the heart muscle itself may become so damaged that even replacement of the valve will not relieve the symptoms.

Mitral Valve Prolapse

Mitral valve prolapse is the most frequently diagnosed cardiac valvular problem—in fact, many physicians feel it is diagnosed far too frequently. The condition affects mostly females and tends to run in families. It is also more common in women who have skeletal abnormalities such as scoliosis (curvature of the spine).

In mitral valve prolapse the leaflets of the mitral valve are more elastic than normal, and they stretch into the left atrium when the ventricle contracts. This may cause no symptoms at all and may be noticed only if a doctor performs echocardiography of the heart valves for some reason. The prolapse sometimes causes a clicking sound, which may be heard through a stethoscope when the heart contracts.

Some persons with mitral valve prolapse have episodes of rapid heartbeat thought to be caused by the valve irritating the heart's pacemaker. About 10 percent of persons with mitral valve prolapse also have some symptoms of mitral regurgitation, but this is almost always very mild. Persons with mitral valve prolapse also have a slight risk of developing infective endocarditis and must take antibiotics before and after dental and surgical procedures.

Aortic Stenosis

Aortic stenosis occurs much more commonly in men than in women, and can occur at almost any age from twenty to sixty. One of the more common causes is a bicuspid aortic valve; that is, the aortic valve has only two, rather than the normal three, leaflets. A bicuspid aortic valve is far more likely to develop calcium deposits leading to aortic stenosis. Other causes include birth defects, the aging process, and perhaps viral infections. A variation, called subaortic stenosis, is caused by enlargement of heart tissue just below the opening of the valve. Even though the valve itself is undamaged, the abnormal tissue obstructs the blood flow through the valve.

When the aortic valve is stenotic, the left ventricle must generate a very high pressure to force blood through the valve and into the blood vessels of the body. Just as the muscles of the body enlarge in a person who constantly lifts weights, the muscular wall of the left ventricle "hypertrophies," becoming very thick. Eventually the muscle can no longer compensate for the narrowing of the valve and cannot pump enough blood to satisfy the body's needs.

At first, the symptoms of aortic stenosis are usually limited to shortness of breath and rapid fatigue during exercise. Eventually, however, all the symptoms of congestive heart failure may develop. Unlike other forms of valvular disease, persons with aortic stenosis are also likely to have fainting spells. The thickened heart muscle requires a very large oxygen supply, but the stenotic valve limits the amount of blood flowing through the coronary arteries to the heart muscle. For this reason, persons with aortic stenosis are also likely to develop angina.

Treatment of aortic stenosis is usually based on the symptoms. In mild cases, limitation of strenuous physical activity, along with prophylactic antibiotics to prevent valve infection, are all that are required. If the disease becomes severe enough to cause angina or symptoms of heart failure at rest, then surgical replacement of the valve is necessary.

Aortic Regurgitation

Aortic regurgitation may occur from a variety of causes. Sometimes persons with bicuspid valves develop regurgitation rather than stenosis. The aortic valve can also be destroyed by infection, or can simply become weak with age. A widening (aneurysm) of the aorta near the valve can also cause aortic regurgitation.

When the aortic valve leaks, blood returns to the left ventricle during diastole, the period when the heart is resting. This blood must be pumped out again, along with the blood that has entered from the left atrium. The left ventricle becomes enlarged to hold the extra blood, and its wall thickens as it is required to pump more blood.

The symptoms of aortic regurgitation include those of congestive failure (fatigue, shortness of breath, fluid retention and swelling) and may also include fainting spells or angina. Persons with aortic regurgitation often have low blood pressure, caused by the inadequate amount of blood flowing from the heart.

As with mitral valve regurgitation, it is sometimes important to replace a regurgitant aortic valve before the symptoms become significant, in order to prevent damage to the heart tissue itself.

Other Valvular Disease

Valvular disease can affect the valves on the right side of the heart (tricuspid and pulmonary valves). Generally, however, stenosis or regurgitation of these valves is tolerated much better than disease involving the valves of the left side of the heart.

Tricuspid stenosis is usually caused either by rheumatic fever or by a congenital defect. When tricuspid stenosis is caused by rheumatic fever, it usually occurs along with aortic or mitral disease. Rarely, it can be caused by a type of cancer called a carcinoid tumor. If symptoms occur from tricuspid stenosis, swelling of the legs and feet is usually present. Fluid retention and pain in the upper right abdomen (caused by swelling of the liver) may also be present.

Tricuspid regurgitation is usually caused by congenital abnormalities, and usually occurs with other congenital cardiac defects. The tricuspid regurgitation itself is usually a small part of the problem in these cases.

Congenital defects are also the most common cause of pulmonary artery stenosis. Less commonly, pulmonary stenosis can be caused by rheumatic fever or tumor. When congenital, pulmonary stenosis is usually part of a number of cardiac abnormalities, and the symptoms vary with the other abnormalities present. Isolated pulmonary stenosis causes symptoms only in severe cases. Fatigue, inability to exercise, and fainting spells may occur.

Pulmonary regurgitation may be caused by endocarditis or by pulmonary hypertension (high blood pressure in the blood vessels of the lungs). Usually there are no symptoms until the right ventricle becomes so enlarged that heart failure occurs. In these cases, the symptoms are similar to those seen with tricuspid regurgitation.

Hypertrophic Subaortic Stenosis

Hypertrophic subaortic stenosis (also known as hypertrophic cardiomyopathy) is not actually a valvular disease but does interfere with blood flow through the aortic valve. In this condition, a section of the heart muscle in the ventricular septum just below the aortic valve becomes so enlarged (hypertrophied) that it interferes with blood flow through the valve.

The cause of the condition is not known, so doctors sometimes refer to it as IHSS (idiopathic hypertrophic subaortic stenosis). It often occurs during the late teens or early twenties and is almost never seen after age thirty-five. It is more common in males than females, and in blacks than whites or Asians.

Because the hypertrophied muscle becomes even larger when the heart contracts strongly, symptoms often occur during exercise. Shortness of breath, chest pain, and fainting during exercise are the most common symptoms seen with this problem. The condition is associated with sudden death, which may occur during strenuous exercise. Medication may relieve symptoms and prevent abnormal heart rhythms, but surgery to remove the muscle mass is necessary for people with severe symptoms.

Congenital Heart Disease

Congenital heart defects usually involve some specific abnormalities of the heart valves, which are discussed above. Although we usually think of heart disease as a problem of middle and old age, 1 of every 200 babies is born with a congenital heart defect. Some of these are so mild that they are not discovered for years, while others cause immediate and severe problems for the infant. The causes of congenital defects are not known with absolute certainty, but most are believed to be a combination of genetics, the environment, and chance.

A couple who has a child with a heart defect is at higher risk than other couples to have future children with heart defects. However, the chances are 95 percent that their future children will be normal. Although most physicians believe that environmental exposures to the fetus may also participate in causing heart defects, no clear evidence has been presented to tell what factors, if any, are important.

The most common heart defects involve abnormal connections between the chambers and large blood vessels of the heart, abnormalities of the heart valves, or abnormalities of the large blood vessels. Discussion of specific congenital heart defects fills up entire books. In all but the most severe cases, however, the condition will either improve on its own or can be surgically corrected. Even very severe heart defects that would have been lethal as recently as the 1980s are being corrected today, sometimes using "in utero" procedures (while the baby is still in the womb).

Monitoring the Severity of Valvular Disease

A physician may suspect the diagnosis of valvular disease from a person's symptoms, history, and physical examination. Routinely, an electrocardiogram is performed to evaluate the conducting system of the heart and to detect any abnormal heart rhythms. (See chapter 7 for more detailed information on specific tests.) A Holter monitor, a computerized electrocardiogram device worn for twenty-four hours a day, may also be ordered to make sure there are no dangerous heart rhythms. Neither of these tests, however, gives much information about the heart valves. Similarly, a chest X ray will detect massive enlargement or pulmonary problems from heart failure, but gives little information about the condition of heart valves.

An echocardiogram is usually performed to evaluate the valves whenever valvular disease is suspected. In echocardiography, ultrasound waves are "bounced" off the surface of the heart, giving a picture of the heart's structure. The test is little different from the ultrasound used to evaluate a fetus in the womb (see chapter 7).

It may also be necessary to perform cardiac catheterization to determine the pressures in the various chambers of the heart. This type of cardiac catheterization is similar to that done for coronary angiography (X-ray studies of the coronary arteries), but slightly different types of catheters are used. Rather than injecting dye, however, a catheter measures the pressure gradient across the valve. The information obtained may give some additional information concerning the degree of valvular disease, but more importantly it can tell the physician a great deal about how well the heart is functioning and whether the heart muscle has been damaged.

After the diagnosis of valvular disease, the condition can often be controlled with medication, at least initially. Once the valves have been damaged, however, the condition tends to worsen with time. It is not unusual for a person to have an infection that causes mild damage to a valve. Decades later, the valve has continued to become more damaged despite the fact that the infection has been gone for many years. Even when valve damage is severe enough to cause symptoms, the heart may be able to compensate for many years.

In general, however, people with significant valvular disease undergo yearly evaluations to determine whether the condition is progressing. These evaluations usually include echocardiography, the use of ultrasound to evaluate the structures of the heart. If the valve reaches a certain degree of abnormality, it will have to be replaced with an artificial valve before irreversible damage to the heart muscle occurs.

Treatment of Valvular Disease

Endocarditis Prophylaxis

Once a heart valve has been damaged even slightly, the person is always at risk for endocarditis. Endocarditis is an infection of the tissue lining the interior of the heart and its valves. If the endocardium is ever damaged, bacteria in a patient's bloodstream can settle onto the endocardium, causing an infection. People with even slight damage to their valves must take antibiotics any time they are even slightly at risk of having bacteria enter their bloodstream. These risks include dental procedures and minor surgical procedures. If endocarditis develops, it will rapidly worsen the valve disease already present.

Medication and Surgery

For many people with mild to moderate valvular heart disease, the symptoms can be controlled with medication to make the heart contract more efficiently or to dilate the blood vessels beyond the diseased valve. Additional medication to remove excess fluid may also be indicated. In some cases, anticoagulants (medication to prevent blood from clotting) may be required. Use of these medications may require monitoring of the blood's clotting ability every month or so. None of the medical treatment corrects the underlying disease, however—it simply alleviates the symptoms so that the affected person can lead a normal life.

Surgery is indicated when medications cannot control the symptoms or if there is risk of permanent damage to the heart muscle or lungs from the valve damage. Depending on the person's age, health, the valve involved, and other considerations, a totally synthetic valve (made of metal and plastic) or a synthetic/animal valve (including animal tissue) may be used.

Chapter 4

HIGH BLOOD
PRESSURE

High blood pressure, or hypertension, is the most common form of heart disease, affecting 60 to 80 million Americans. It is one of the most common causes of heart failure and heart attacks, as well as strokes and kidney failure. Unfortunately, high blood pressure by itself causes few, if any, symptoms. It is only detected if a person's blood pressure is checked regularly.

The likelihood of having high blood pressure is proportional to age. Less than 5 percent of thirty-year-olds have high blood pressure, while 40 percent of persons over age sixty-five have some degree of hypertension.

Before 1970, only half of the people with high blood pressure were even aware that they had the condition, and only half of those who knew received adequate treatment. As late as 1990, 25 percent of people with high blood pressure did not know they had the condition, and one-third of those who did know were not receiving adequate treatment.

What Is High Blood Pressure?

As the heart pumps blood out, pressure is created by the resistance of the arteries. This pressure can be measured easily using a sphygmomanometer (blood pressure cuff and measuring devices). Blood pressure readings are given in two numbers, such as 130/75. The numbers represent millimeters of mercury, often abbreviated mm Hg. The original sphygmomanometers contained a column of mercury that acted as a weight on the blood pressure cuff. The reading represented how high the column was when the pressure of the blood forced it through the cuff.

The first number measures the pressure generated when the heart is pumping (systole), while the second measures the pressure between contractions (diastole). Although the average blood pressure reading for adults is usually stated to be 120/80, a slightly higher or lower reading can still be considered normal.

Recently new information has become available about what levels of blood pressure are safe. Historically, the diastolic (lower number) blood pressure was considered to be the most important, and medical treatment was only considered necessary if the diastolic pressure was greater than 95. Elevations of just the systolic (upper number) alone were not considered to be significant, and mild high blood pressure in older persons was considered normal.

Today, the upper limit of normal is considered to be 140/90 for people over forty-five years of age, although a person may have a higher reading once in a while. For people under forty-five, 130/90 is considered the upper limit of normal. A person whose blood pressure is usually higher than this is considered to have hypertension. These levels were not decided arbitrarily. They were determined by large clinical studies that showed that people with blood pressures higher than these levels were 50 percent more likely to die from complications of hypertension than were other people of similar age.

Several large studies published in the early and mid-1990s demonstrated that the systolic pressure (the top reading) could be as important as the diastolic reading. Even a moderately elevated systolic pressure (greater than 140) increases a person's chance of developing heart disease and stroke. The National Heart, Lung, and Blood Institute (NHLBI) coined the term *isolated systolic hypertension* (ISH) for this condition. These studies also found that ISH in the elderly was just as dangerous as it was in younger people. Today it is recommended that any person with a systolic pressure consistently above 140, or a diastolic pressure above 90, begin medical treatment for hypertension.

What Causes High Blood Pressure?

In some cases, a disease causes hypertension as one of its effects. Kidney disease is among the more common causes, as are some hormonal abnormalities. Some drugs, including amphetamines (even the ones found in cold pills), cocaine, birth control pills, and steroids can also cause hypertension. This kind of high blood pressure is referred to as secondary hypertension, and it can be cured by treating the original medical problem. Secondary hypertension accounts for only about 5 percent of all cases of high blood pressure.

Most cases of hypertension have no specific known cause; these are called essential or primary hypertension. Some factors definitely increase a person's risk of developing high blood pressure, however. There is a genetic component—high blood pressure runs in families. It is also more common, and tends to be more severe, in blacks than in whites or Asians. Other possible risk factors include obesity, diets high in salt, and chronic stress.

We also know that some abnormalities occur in many people with high blood pressure. The body contains several hormonal systems to regulate blood pressure. The most important is the renin-angiotensin-aldosterone system. This is a group of hormonal messengers that tell the kidneys to retain fluid and the blood vessels to contract. This system is abnormal in some, but not all, persons with primary hypertension. Several other hormonal systems are also active in blood pressure control. It is likely that abnormalities in any of several regulating mechanisms could lead to hypertension.

The Signs and Symptoms of High Blood Pressure

High blood pressure generally causes no symptoms, or at most results in headaches. Inside the body, however, it steadily causes damage to several organs and tissues. The kidneys are very sensitive to high blood pressure, and hypertension is one of the most common causes of kidney failure. It is also a significant cause of stroke (bleeding or blood clots in the brain).

High blood pressure also results in several forms of heart disease, including hypertrophic cardiomyopathy, coronary artery disease, and (eventually) congestive heart failure. Hypertension becomes even more important when a person develops heart disease. When the heart attempts to force blood against a higher blood pressure, its workload increases dramatically. This can rapidly worsen congestive heart failure and makes a person with coronary artery disease much more likely to have a heart attack.

Treatment of High Blood Pressure

Hypertension can usually be controlled easily by a combination of medications and changes in daily habits. The severity of an individual's hypertension, as well as the presence of other medical problems, determines which treatment is best. People with mild hypertension can sometimes return their blood pressure to normal levels simply by losing weight, eating less salt, reducing alcohol intake, and exercising. Seventy percent of persons who follow these recommendations can stop taking blood pressure medications by making these lifestyle changes.

Weight loss and exercise benefit every hypertensive patient. It is important that both the exercise program and the diet be approved by a doctor. Overvigorous exercise in a person with hypertension or other heart disease can be dangerous, especially if coronary disease or any degree of heart failure is present. A sensible exercise program will show dramatic benefits within three months.

It has long been recommended that all hypertensive patients avoid sodium (table salt). In more recent years it has been shown that this is particularly important for black persons with hypertension. It has also been shown that supplemental potassium (an ingredient in many salt substitutes), calcium, and magnesium may have a beneficial effect in reducing blood pressure, at least for some patients. The benefits of these supplements have been demonstrated in only a few studies, however. They may also have harmful effects for certain people, especially if taken in high doses. Check with your doctor before taking these supplements, especially magnesium.

Persons with more severe hypertension generally require medical therapy. Many people are under the impression that blood pressure medication causes a lot of side effects. In the past, this was true—male impotence, depression, fatigue, and dizziness occurred with many of the blood pressure medications. Today, however, there are so many effective medications for treating hypertension that almost everyone can find an effective medication without side effects. Unfortunately, there is no cure for hypertension, so medication may be required for the rest of the affected person's life, especially if the hypertension is severe. It is very important that patients do not stop taking blood pressure medication on their own, even if they have made major lifestyle changes. Some people have dramatically increased blood pressure when they stop their medication even for a few days. This can result in bleeding within the brain (cerebral hemorrhage), sudden heart failure, or heart attack.

Medical treatment of high blood pressure (see chapter 8) usually begins with a diuretic drug, which may be all that is required. If the hypertension is more severe, other drugs may be added. In many cases it takes a bit of trial and error to select the right medicines, since every person responds differently to different drugs. In almost every case, however, effective control of blood pressure can be obtained with minimal side effects.

Chapter 5

CONGESTIVE HEART FAILURE AND CARDIOMYOPATHY

Congestive Heart Failure

Heart failure simply means that the heart is not pumping enough blood to meet all the body's needs. Because one of the first symptoms is the retention of fluid in the tissues, or "congestion," it is often referred to as congestive heart failure. Heart failure affects about 1 percent of all adults in the United States at any given time. While heart failure is always a serious condition, it has many degrees of severity and often can be corrected. It is important to remember that the term *heart failure* refers to an end result. Many different types of heart disease can eventually cause heart failure if they become severe enough. The outcome and treatment of heart failure often depend more on what the underlying disease is than on how severe the heart failure is.

Symptoms of Congestive Heart Failure

All the symptoms of heart failure result from inability of the heart to pump enough blood to the tissues and backup of blood into the veins (sometimes called venous congestion), which allows fluid to collect in the organs and tissues of the body (edema).

With mild degrees of heart failure there may be only a mild swelling around the ankles and some shortness of breath during exertion. As heart failure worsens, more fluid retention occurs, leading to swelling in the legs and hands. Fluid retention in the lungs can cause orthopnea, shortness of breath when lying flat. For this reason persons with congestive heart failure often sleep on several pillows, or with the head of their bed propped up. Inadequate blood flow to the body results in shortness of breath with even mild exertion, such as walking across a room.

In the most severe cases, congestive heart failure causes shortness of breath even at rest. The arms and legs become cool and pale from lack of blood flow, and cyanosis (bluish color) may be seen in the lips and fingernails from lack of oxygen in the blood. Cheyne-Stokes respiration, which is a pattern of alternating slow deep breathing, pauses, and rapid breathing, may develop. Blood flow to the kidneys is reduced, resulting in further fluid accumulation.

Sometimes, lying down for an extended period of time allows even more fluid to accumulate in the lungs. This often occurs in the middle of the night after several hours' sleep, causing the affected person to wake up very short of breath. This is referred to as paroxysmal nocturnal dyspnea, which simply means sudden shortness of breath in the middle of the night.

If one side of the heart is in more severe failure than the other, it may be referred to as "right-sided" or "left-sided" heart failure. Left-sided failure causes blood to back up in the lungs, so shortness of breath and orthopnea are the most prominent symptoms. When left-sided failure is severe, pulmonary edema (fluid filling the lungs) can result. Right-sided failure causes more swelling of the extremities. In severe cases the liver and internal organs also swell, causing bloating and abdominal discomfort.

Causes of Heart Failure

Heart failure occurs when any form of heart disease has progressed to the point that the heart can no longer pump blood adequately. One of the most common causes of congestive heart failure is coronary artery disease and resulting heart attacks that have damaged or destroyed a significant amount of heart muscle. Inadequately treated high blood pressure is another common cause. Valvular heart disease, severe lung problems, and cardiomyopathy can also result in congestive heart failure.

Treatment of Congestive Heart Failure

When a treatable underlying cause of congestive failure exists, correcting the cause may resolve, or at least greatly improve, the degree of heart failure (see chapter 8 for more information). For example, replacing a diseased valve may completely resolve the symptoms of congestive failure. If significant coronary artery disease is present, restoring adequate circulation to the heart can greatly improve the ability of the heart muscle to contract. Congestive heart failure caused by hypertension may improve markedly when the blood pressure is brought back to normal.

Even when there is no treatable cause of congestive failure, medical therapy can markedly improve the symptoms. Medical therapy generally has five goals:

1. Improve the contracting ability of the heart.
2. Remove excess sodium (salt) and fluid from the body.

3. Reduce the amount of work the heart must do to pump blood.

4. Restore a normal heart rhythm

5. Prevent blood clots from forming (thromboembolism).

Several types of medication can improve contraction of the heart. As a group they are called inotropes. The digitalis class of drugs has been used effectively for this purpose for well over a century and remains the most commonly used medication today. In some persons, however, the inotropes increase the workload of the heart and may not be appropriate.

Excessive fluid and salt can usually be removed by diuretic medications. A host of diuretics are available, and proper selection depends on the severity of the patient's heart failure and the condition of the kidneys, as well as other individual variations between people. It often takes trials of two or three diuretics before the best one for a given individual is determined.

Reducing the workload on the heart is accomplished by vasodilators, medications that dilate the blood vessels and thus allow blood to flow forward with lower pressures. Many different types of vasodilators may be used, including antihypertensives and nitroglycerin type drugs. Angiotensin converting enzyme (ACE) inhibitors are also used frequently because they work to decrease levels of a vasoconstricting hormone that becomes elevated in congestive heart failure.

Medication to prevent blood clots (anticoagulants) is not always required. In many cases a low dose of aspirin, which inhibits platelet clotting, is all that is required. A few people may need stronger anticoagulants (often referred to as blood thinners). Medication to restore heart rhythm is needed in only a few cases.

In a few cases, surgery may be indicated to treat congestive failure. If abnormal heart rhythm contributes to the congestive failure, a pacemaker may help to restore normal rhythm (see chapter 11). In the most severe cases, the patient may be considered as a heart transplant candidate (see chapter 9). While artificial hearts are inadequate for long-term use, ventricular assist devices are sometimes used to temporarily help the ventricle to pump if there is hope that the heart may heal over a period of a week or so.

Two new (and at this time still experimental) procedures also hold out some hope for helping persons with congestive heart failure (see chapter 15). One involves surgical removal of the most diseased parts of the ventricle, in hopes that the remaining healthier tissue will then be able to pump more effectively. The other involves removal of healthy muscle tissue from the inside of the back; the tissue is then wrapped around the heart. A pacemaker is used to make this healthy tissue contract, assisting the heart muscle as it pumps.

Cardiomyopathy

Cardiomyopathy, which literally means "disease of the heart muscle," is a group of heart diseases that have congestive heart failure as their major symptom. Cardiomyopathies are not common; taken together, all cardiomyopathies account for only 1 percent of all cardiac deaths in the United States. They are important, however, because they can be so severe.

The several types of cardiomyopathy may be labeled either by their cause (if known) or by a description of their symptoms. This can create some confusion, since the same disease may be referred to by more than one name. For example, excessive alcohol intake can cause a cardiomyopathy that dilates the heart. It may be referred to by its cause (alcoholic cardiomyopathy), or by its anatomic description (dilated cardiomyopathy).

Even worse, doctors often use the term *enlarged heart* when talking to patients about cardiomyopathy. This is really no more useful than saying "something is wrong." It can refer to dilated cardiomyopathy (a condition in which the heart's chambers are enlarged from muscle weakness); to a heart that is dilated from another form of congestive heart failure; to a heart with thickened walls from hypertrophic (enlarged muscle) cardiomyopathy or hypertension; or to a heart that is enlarged from problems in the lungs.

In this book, we will refer to the cardiomyopathies primarily by their anatomically descriptive names for the sake of simplicity. For most cases of cardiomyopathy, the cause is unknown (idiopathic) anyway. I will avoid the term *enlarged heart*.

Anatomically, cardiomyopathy can be grouped into three major categories:

1. Dilated cardiomyopathy, in which the heart muscle becomes thin and weak, resulting in enlargement of the heart's chambers.
2. Hypertrophic cardiomyopathy, in which the heart muscle becomes very thick and overgrown.
3. Restrictive cardiomyopathy, in which the heart becomes stiff and has difficulty filling with blood.

Dilated Cardiomyopathy

Dilated cardiomyopathy begins when the heart is unable to contract efficiently and only a small portion of the blood in the ventricles is ejected with each heartbeat. As more blood remains in the ventricles after contraction, they overfill and become larger. In some ways, this is a built-in compensation mechanism that the heart uses to maintain blood flow. The ventricle normally contains about 150 milliliters (ml) of blood and ejects 60 percent (90 ml) with each beat. If the heart can only eject 30 percent, it will begin to dilate. Once the volume in the ventricle reaches 300 ml, ejecting only 30 percent will still provide 90 ml of blood to the body with each heartbeat.

Unfortunately, this compensation only works to a point. After the heart has enlarged to a certain degree, it becomes unable to pump as efficiently, and the amount of blood ejected decreases further. Because the valves are attached to the heart muscle, extreme dilation may make the valves leak, worsening the heart's ability to pump blood.

Many cases of dilated cardiomyopathy are idiopathic. Some of these cases are associated with inflammation of the heart muscle, leading many researchers to believe that a viral illness may be the cause. Idiopathic cardiomyopathy can occur at any age; men are more likely to be affected than women.

Dilated cardiomyopathy may also be caused by toxic chemicals, including long-term alcohol abuse, some cancer chemotherapy drugs, and exposure to a few toxic chemicals such as beryllium. It can also be caused by severe nutritional abnormalities and vitamin deficiencies. A few cases occur during pregnancy or in association with some rare neurologic disorders. There is also a genetic form that tends to run in a few families.

The symptoms of dilated cardiomyopathy are the same as those of congestive heart failure. Dilated cardiomyopathy is quite serious, and as many as half the people affected with it die within one year. In recent years, treatment of the condition has become more effective, however. Medical therapy to remove excess fluid, reduce the workload of the heart, and improve the heart's ability to pump can markedly reduce symptoms, often for many years. When medical treatment is ineffective, heart transplantation may be the only alternative.

Hypertrophic Cardiomyopathy

Hypertrophic cardiomyopathy is much less common than dilated cardiomyopathy. The most common form, idiopathic hypertrophic subaortic stenosis (IHSS), is discussed as one of the valvular heart diseases (see chapter 3), since its symptoms resemble those of aortic stenosis. Generalized hypertrophy of the heart muscle causes problems because the heart is unable to fill with blood properly.

Hypertrophic cardiomyopathy may result from years of high blood pressure or from untreated valvular stenosis, but sometimes it is idiopathic. A genetic form that runs in families also occurs. The condition can occur as early as the twenties, although the type caused by hypertension may not occur until middle age.

The most striking symptom of hypertrophic cardiomyopathy is fainting or dizziness with exertion. Chest pain, shortness of breath, palpitations (episodes of rapid heartbeat), and the symptoms of congestive heart failure also occur. Hypertrophic cardiomyopathy is not as deadly as dilated cardiomyopathy, but about 3 percent of the people with this condition will die within one year, usually suddenly. Luckily, in the majority of people who have hypertrophic cardiomyopathy the disease does not progress. Medical treatment can relieve some of the symptoms and protect against irregular heartbeats.

Restrictive Cardiomyopathy

Restrictive cardiomyopathy is fairly rare. In this form of cardiomyopathy, the heart is usually of normal size but cannot expand to fill with blood properly. Even though the contracting power of the heart is often normal in restrictive cardiomyopathy, it cannot pump out sufficient amounts of blood because it cannot fill with blood efficiently.

A few diseases are known to cause restrictive cardiomyopathy. Connective tissue diseases, especially scleroderma, may cause the heart muscle to be replaced by fibrous tissue, causing restrictive cardiomyopathy. Reaction to a few drugs can cause a similar effect. Amyloidosis (a rare condition in which excessive protein is deposited in various tissues of the body) and hemochromatosis (a similar condition in which excessive iron is deposited in the tissues) can also cause restrictive cardiomyopathy. Occasionally the pericardium (the sac of connective tissue that contains the heart) becomes infected or inflamed, causing restriction of the heart's filling, even though the heart muscle itself is normal.

Most causes of restrictive cardiomyopathy are idiopathic, however. Idiopathic restrictive cardiomyopathy usually occurs in the fifties or sixties and affects men and women equally. Few effective medical treatments exist, and heart transplantation is sometimes required.

Chapter 6

RHYTHM DISTURBANCES

Abnormal heartbeats are called dysrhythmias, meaning abnormal rhythms (older books may refer to them as arrhythmias, which actually means "no rhythm"). Whenever any part of the heart's conducting system is damaged, a dysrhythmia can result. Such conducting system damage may result from a heart attack, from chemical or nutritional abnormalities, a genetic defect, or simply from the aging process. In the majority of cases, the dysrhythmias result from some other type of heart disease, usually heart attack.

The signs of dysrhythmias range in severity from no symptoms at all, to occasional episodes of rapid heartbeat or a "skipped" heartbeat, through fainting spells, to complete cardiac arrest. In many cases dysrhythmias are detected on a routine electrocardiogram in people who had no indication of a problem. Dysrhythmias are fairly common, affecting about 6.5 million Americans.

Unlike other forms of heart disease, dysrhythmias do not usually worsen over time. A person who has one type of dysrhythmia with minimal symptoms is not likely to progress to a more severe dysrhythmia over time.

Conduction Defects

Dysrhythmias are broadly grouped into two types: conduction defects and abnormal pacemakers. Conduction defects occur when some part of the electrical conducting system of the heart is damaged. If the damage occurs between the sinus node and the atrioventricular node (see Figure 1-5), the resulting dysrhythmia is called heart block or atrioventricular block, since the beats originate properly but are blocked from reaching the most important parts of the heart—the ventricles.

Heart block does not usually completely block the impulse from reaching the ventricles, but it interferes with its conduction to some degree. Heart block is classified according to the degree of severity. Grade I heart block results only in a delay of the beat's conduction and has little clinical significance. As a general rule it causes no symptoms and needs no treatment, other than an EKG every six months to twelve months to make sure it doesn't get any worse. Grade II heart block not only delays the conduction of the heartbeat to the ventricle, but also causes an occasional beat to be dropped completely. Some types of grade II heart block can be tolerated and require no treatment, while others require medication or the insertion of a pacemaker.

In grade III heart block, no beats are conducted from the sinus node to the atrioventricular node. Usually, the atrioventricular node will take over the pacemaking function to some degree, sending impulses to the ventricle on its own. These atrioventricular beats occur less frequently than the normal sinus impulses, however, resulting in a very slow pulse. Almost every person with grade III heart block will require a pacemaker.

Heart block can also occur in the conducting system below the atrioventricular node. In this case it results from damage to the bundles of conducting fibers between the node and the ventricles. This type of heart block is referred to as a bundle branch block. Depending on which of the actual bundles are affected (this can be determined by an EKG), it may be called a "right" or "left" bundle branch block. Additionally, the left bundle splits into two separate branches. Some left bundle branch blocks affect only one of the branches; these are referred to as left bundle branch hemiblock.

When bundle branch block occurs, the impulse moves normally through the unaffected part of the conducting system to the heart muscle, which contracts normally. The impulse is also passed slowly through the heart muscle and then is conducted backward through the damaged bundle (Figure 6-1). This is referred to as retrograde (backward) conduction.

When retrograde conduction occurs, part of the heart contracts normally with the beat, while the "blocked" area of the heart contracts later and in a less coordinated fashion via the retrograde conduction. While this does allow the affected ventricle to contract, it interferes with the coordination of the heartbeat, and the heart does not pump as efficiently as it normally does.

Generally bundle branch blocks do not cause significant symptoms, but sometimes they predispose patients to episodes of extremely rapid heartbeat, called ventricular tachycardia. This can occur with some bundle branch blocks by a mechanism called impulse reentry. Impulse reentry occurs when the delayed impulse caused by retrograde conduction reenters the main conducting system of the heart, causing an abnormal heartbeat that originates in the ventricles. Often this results in a situation where one normal heartbeat is immediately followed by a second, abnormal beat—a condition called bigeminy. This may cause few problems but sometimes interferes with the heart's pumping ability.

In a few cases, impulse reentry results in a series of very rapid heartbeats known as ventricular tachycardia. This is a very severe dysrhythmia, interfering with the heart's ability to pump blood and even causing cardiac arrest. An episode of ventricular tachycardia is usually considered a medical emergency.

Abnormal Pacemakers

Abnormal pacemakers result when some part of the heart other than one of the nodes begins to send out electrical contraction signals. It is believed that abnormal pacemakers usually originate from heart tissue that is damaged but not totally destroyed. The damaged cells become "leaky" to the charged ions in the fluid around them, resulting in periodic electrical discharges that start a contraction. These abnormal pacemakers usually originate from cells in the ventricles and are called premature ventricular contractions, or PVCs.

The occurrence of a few PVCs is nothing to be worried about. Almost everyone will have one once in a while. People with heart disease often have frequent PVCs, however, as many as several a minute. Although PVCs cause the heart to contract, they usually pump less blood than a normal beat, since their contraction is not coordinated properly by the conducting system. More importantly, PVCs sometimes can start reentry beats, resulting in ventricular tachycardia, a series of abnormal beats.

Ventricular tachycardia causes such rapid beats that the heart cannot fill with blood properly and cannot pump out enough blood to supply the organs of the body. At the same time, the heart is working very hard and using a lot of oxygen. If the person having ventricular tachycardia has coronary artery disease, a heart attack is likely to occur. If ventricular tachycardia continues for more than a few minutes, it can become a life-threatening emergency.

If the beats become totally uncoordinated, the heart no longer contracts as a unit, but rather each of the individual myocytes contracts on its own. This is known as ventricular fibrillation. When a heart in ventricular fibrillation is observed, it appears to quiver and does not pump blood at all. For all practical purposes, a fibrillating heart has stopped completely, and cardiopulmonary resuscitation (CPR) must be started. Defibrillation, using direct current shocks to stop the fibrillating, is used in the hope that a normal heartbeat will begin.

Treatment of PVCs is necessary if they are frequent enough to interfere with the heart's pumping action, or if there is a risk that they may cause ventricular tachycardia or ventricular fibrillation. Medications can reduce the number of PVCs, as well as the risk of more lethal dysrhythmias. Medications may also increase the risk of sudden death in patients with PVCs, however, and should be used only when a patient is at major risk. Reduction of caffeine, alcohol, and over-the-counter medications (especially cold pills) can dramatically reduce the frequency of PVCs. In a few cases, an implanted device similar to a pacemaker is used to defibrillate the heart automatically if ventricular tachycardia or fibrillation occurs.

It is also possible for the heart's normal pacemakers to become damaged and fail to function properly. Pacemaker abnormalities usually involve the sinus node. If the sinus node becomes damaged, it may send very rapid electrical signals to the heart. This causes sinus tachycardia, a series of very rapid heartbeats originating from the sinus node. The condition can be similar to ventricular tachycardia, but in most cases the atrioventricular node blocks some of the rapid beats, protecting the ventricles from beating too rapidly.

Alternatively, a damaged sinus node may cause atrial fibrillation, uncoordinated twitching of the atrial myocytes. In atrial fibrillation the atrioventricular node assumes the pacemaker function for the ventricles, maintaining a normal heartbeat and pulse. The heart's pumping effectiveness is decreased by about 10 percent when atrial fibrillation occurs, however. Sinus dysrhythmias are usually treated with medications, but occasionally a pacemaker is required.

Diagnosis of Dysrhythmias

When a person is believed to have a dysrhythmia, either because of symptoms or because a doctor feels abnormal beats when taking a pulse, a routine series of tests is performed (see also chapter 7). An EKG may be all that is necessary to diagnose the dysrhythmia, but since an EKG observes the heart only for a few minutes, it may not show the complete range of abnormal beats. A Holter cardiac monitor may be used to show a more complete picture. This consists of wearing a portable, battery-powered EKG machine for an entire day. The machine stores the entire day's EKG readings, and later downloads the information into a computer for analysis.

In rare cases, a rhythm disturbance may be so severe that medical therapy cannot control the abnormal beats and surgery to remove the abnormal pacemaker or conducting system is needed. To localize the abnormal tissue, a form of cardiac catheterization may be used. The catheter used in this instance contains an EKG electrode in its tip, which can localize the abnormality very accurately.

Section II

EVALUATING
AND TREATING
HEART DISEASE

Chapter 7

DIAGNOSIS AND MONITORING OF HEART DISEASE

Probably no area of medicine has advanced as much in the past twenty-five years as the evaluation of heart disease. The evaluation may seem greatly different in different circumstances—a person in the midst of a heart attack is treated quite differently than one who occasionally has some shortness of breath during exertion, for example. While the circumstances differ greatly, the tests performed are basically the same.

As diagnostic tests, especially invasive tests (those that require putting a needle or catheter into the body), have become more sophisticated they have in some cases developed into treatments. The most striking example is a patient who has a cardiac catheterization to examine the coronary arteries and at the same time undergoes angioplasty to correct any blockage.

The Preliminary Examination

It is probably the preliminary examination that varies most with circumstances. It may take only seconds for a doctor to realize that someone is in extreme heart failure, but it may take a lengthy examination to determine whether an occasional chest pain is truly a symptom of mild angina.

In nonemergency situations (and to some degree even in emergencies), the patient's history is the most important part of the evaluation. Invasive cardiac tests are expensive, time-consuming, and carry some slight risk to the patient. No physician wants to order them unnecessarily, so a detailed history of the problem is taken to determine whether further tests are needed.

Patients sometimes become frustrated by a doctor who spends a lot of time asking about their symptoms, but this usually indicates an excellent physician. An experienced physician can often get a good idea of the type and severity of heart disease just by listening to the person describe the symptoms.

The history usually begins by evaluation of cardiac risk factors, which determine how likely a person is to have heart disease (see chapter 12). A family history of heart problems, male gender, age over fifty-five, high blood pressure, a history of high blood cholesterol, and a high-stress/low-exercise lifestyle all make it more likely that a person has heart disease.

The physical examination involves examining the hands, feet, and neck for signs of venous congestion, indicating the heart is not pumping well. Use of a stethoscope to listen to the chest can sometimes indicate whether excess fluid is accumulating in the lungs from congestive heart failure. Listening to the heartbeat can reveal abnormal sounds caused by valvular disease or pericarditis (inflammation of the lining around the heart), and abnormal heartbeats caused by dysrhythmia. Listening over various blood vessels may reveal a swishing sound (called a bruit) that could indicate obstruction from atherosclerosis.

Taking the blood pressure may show hypertension, but a single high blood pressure reading does not mean the patient has hypertension.

Physicians often refer to "white-coat hypertension," a falsely high reading that is the result of anxiety and nervousness from being in the doctor's office. If a high reading is obtained, the doctor will probably have the blood pressure retaken several times over several days or weeks to see if it truly remains above normal.

Routine Tests

Blood Tests

If you have not had a physical examination in a while, the preliminary examination may include some blood tests. Most of the time an automated battery of tests is run, including counts of red and white blood cells as well as the different electrolytes and chemicals in the blood. These tests often report back on twenty-four or twenty-six different analyses of the blood. It is not unusual to have one or more "abnormal" results, since these tests simply compare the levels in your blood to what is considered average. A pattern of several related tests being abnormal, or of one or two tests being far from the normal range, may be a cause of concern.

Most people being evaluated for possible heart disease will also undergo a lipid profile, an analysis of the lipids (fats) in the blood. An accurate lipid profile requires that you not eat for six to twelve hours prior to the test, since food intake will elevate the triglyceride level (but not the cholesterol). Usually four substances are analyzed: triglycerides, cholesterol, low-density lipoprotein (LDL), and high-density lipoprotein (HDL).

All the lipid profile numbers are important, but they can be confusing. The simplest analysis is to look at total cholesterol. Several studies followed thousands of people for years to determine if there was a link between cholesterol levels and heart attack. All have found that the higher the cholesterol, the higher the risk of heart attack. For example, one study showed that people with cholesterol levels over 300 were four

Table 7-1: Lipid Profile and Heart Attack Risk

	Good	Slight Risk	High Risk
Total Cholesterol	<200	200–239	>240
LDL Cholesterol	<130	130–159	>160
LDL / HDL ratio	<3	3–5	>5
HDL Cholesterol	>45	35–45	<35

times as likely to have a heart attack as people with cholesterol levels under 180. It has also been shown that lowering cholesterol levels 10 percent results in a 20 percent decrease in heart attack risk.

It is a little more accurate to look at the two types of cholesterol separately, however. You may have heard of "good" cholesterol and "bad" cholesterol. This is because LDL cholesterol tends to put fat into the arteries of people with atherosclerosis. HDL cholesterol carries cholesterol to the liver, where it can be metabolized into substances the body needs. The level of LDL cholesterol and the ratio of LDL to HDL are also important in determining heart attack risk (see Table 7-1). Notice that the more HDL cholesterol, the *lower* the heart attack risk.

If it is suspected that you may have had a heart attack, cardiac enzyme tests may be ordered. These analyze the blood to see whether it contains any of a few enzymes that normally exist only in the heart. If they are found in the blood, it indicates that heart cells have died, releasing their contents into the bloodstream. If the enzymes are found, their concentration is roughly proportional to the amount of heart muscle that has been damaged.

The cardiac enzymes usually analyzed for are creatinine kinase (CK) and lactate dehydrogenase (LDH). Varieties of these two enzymes are found in many other tissues of the body and grossly analyzed for on the blood-test battery mentioned above. Only analysis for the specific types of CK and LDH found in heart tissue can indicate a heart attack.

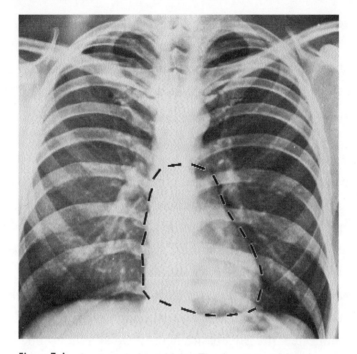

Figure 7-1: *A normal chest X ray. The heart is outlined.*

Chest X Rays

Everyone knows that chest X rays show the internal structure of the chest, but some people falsely believe that they give a detailed view of the heart and lungs. An actual chest X ray is rather shadowy (Figure 7-1). It provides a lot of general information, but not a lot of specific information about heart disease.

Although none of the particular structures of the heart show up on a chest X ray, the X ray clearly shows the overall shape and size of the heart. An X ray is the simplest way to determine whether there is cardiac enlargement from dilation or hypertrophy of the heart, but it does not clearly show which of the two conditions is causing the enlargement. Evaluation of the lungs may also show whether fluid is accumulating in them, but not the cause. Overall, then, the chest X ray can demonstrate whether significant heart failure is present.

In a few cases it may also show calcification (formation of calcium deposits in the tissues). This may occur when tissue has been injured or damaged for a long time. Some persons with valvular heart disease will have calcified valves that are visible on X ray, and a very few persons have calcified coronary arteries or calcifications in the aorta.

Electrocardiogram (EKG)

Every patient with the symptoms of heart disease should get an electrocardiogram. When the heart muscle contracts, electrically charged ions (small atoms such as sodium or potassium) enter and leave the muscle cells. The movement of these ions generates a very small electrical current. An EKG is a device to measure that current.

The EKG machine is connected to your body by several sticky pads that are coated with a conducting gel. Although as many as twelve pads may be connected, the EKG basically uses two at a time—one positive and one negative electrode. By altering which of the electrodes the EKG uses for each reading, it can "look" at the electrical activity of the heart from several directions. Each of these directions is referred to as a "lead." Usually the printed EKG contains twelve leads, providing electrical views of the heart from several directions.

Depending on which lead is being used, the EKG tracing may look slightly different (Figure 7-2). The tracing usually has the same constant features in each lead, although they may have different proportions and shapes depending on the lead selected. The small P wave shows the contraction of the atria. The larger QRS complex shows the contraction of the ventricles. The T wave is formed as the heart repolarizes, getting ready for the next beat.

The EKG shows the heart's rate and rhythm. Whenever a rhythm disturbance is present, the normal structure of the EKG waves is altered. In a conduction defect, for example, the P waves and QRS complexes do not follow one another properly. Beats originating from abnormal pace-

makers will have dramatically abnormal shapes (Figure 7-2).

The EKG sometimes (but not
always) will be abnormal during a
heart attack, or even years after a
person has recovered from a heart
attack. Elevation of the region
between the QRS complex or re-
versal of the T wave itself may indicate that the heart is not getting
enough blood or that a heart attack is occurring. Years after a
heart attack, there may be a deep
cleft at the start of the QRS complex. Sometimes, by seeing which
lead the changes have occurred in,
the cardiologist can determine
roughly what part of the heart is
affected. At other times the EKG
may appear perfectly normal even
though a person is having a severe
heart attack.

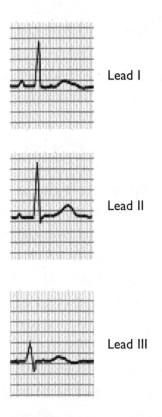

Lead I

Lead II

Lead III

Figure 7-2: *An EKG tracing of a single heartbeat showing differences and similarities from three different leads.*

As mentioned in other chapters, a twenty-four-hour EKG (also called a Holter monitor) may be used to evaluate the heart over a longer period of time. This involves wearing a portable EKG unit that records the entire day's activities of the heart. The data are then fed into a computer that analyzes the total number of abnormal beats. A physician can then analyze the beats further. Patients are usually asked to record activities and symptoms in a notebook while wearing the monitor, so that the physician can correlate the abnormal beats with these events.

Less commonly, an event-recording EKG may be used. This is a similar device, but rather than recording the entire day's heartbeats, it only records when the patient has a symptom and pushes a button on the device. It is useful in cases when symptoms occur only every few days.

Noninvasive Tests of the Heart and Blood Vessels

Noninvasive tests are those that don't require any testing equipment to actually enter your body, although in a few cases you may receive an injection as part of the test. Noninvasive tests generally have lower complication rates, since you are not exposed to infection or possible damage to your tissues. For this reason, noninvasive tests are preferred whenever possible.

Exercise Electrocardiogram

The exercise electrocardiogram is often referred to as a treadmill or stress test. Its purpose is to use exercise (usually walking on a treadmill or riding a stationary bicycle) to stress the heart by increasing the amount of blood it must pump. The heart usually has enormous reserves and can compensate for many forms of heart disease while the body is resting. With exercise it must work harder, and any disease symptoms are more likely to be revealed.

The EKG used in a stress test is no different from a normal EKG. It is monitored while you walk on a treadmill, and every few minutes the inclination (slope) of the treadmill is made steeper to increase the amount of exercise. Since everyone is in different shape, the doctors performing the test constantly ask how hard the exercise seems for you. They also monitor your heart rate, since there is a good correlation between the rate and how hard the heart is working. The test is stopped when you reach your exercise limit, when your heart rate reaches what is considered maximum for your age, or when you feel any chest pain or when symptoms of heart problems show up on the EKG.

EKG stress tests are not very dangerous, but there is a small chance of a patient having a heart attack during the strenuous exercise. This would only occur, however, in a person who had coronary artery disease and was likely to have a heart attack soon anyway. A cardiologist is always immediately available whenever a stress test is performed.

A normal exercise EKG does not absolutely mean that there is no heart disease present. It does give strong indication that there is no severe coronary artery disease, however, and usually it means that no further testing is needed for a year or so. In rare cases the stress test can be normal despite coronary disease. If a doctor feels strongly from the patient's history that coronary disease is present, further tests may be ordered despite a normal exercise EKG.

Nuclear Medicine Scans

In nuclear medicine scans, a tiny amount of mildly radioactive chemical is injected inside the body, and then a cameralike detector outside the body tracks where the chemical goes and provides a computer-enhanced picture. Different radioactive chemicals are used depending on what the physician wants a picture of. Some remain in the bloodstream and can provide information about how the heart is pumping. Others enter the heart muscle and show how it is working and what the coronary circulation is like. Others can provide a picture of the circulation of the lungs.

The nuclear medicine scan performed most commonly for assessing heart disease is called radionuclide ventriculography (meaning radioactive chemical picture of the ventricles). It can also be referred to as a MUGA scan, for multi-gated acquisition. To perform the test, a chemical (usually technetium, so the test is often called a technetium scan) is injected into the bloodstream through a vein in the arm.

The technetium binds to the red blood cells, so it remains in the circulatory system. As it passes through the heart, the detecting cameras show the size and shape of the ventricles. The scan also gives numerical evidence of the volume of blood contained in the ventricles and how much is ejected with each heartbeat. A technetium scan can also be studied to see if all parts of the ventricle are working equally well. If part of the heart muscle in the ventricular wall has an insufficient blood supply or is scarred from an old heart attack, it won't move as much as the rest of the ventricle during a contraction.

A MUGA scan may also be performed as you exercise, in a fashion similar to an exercise EKG. Scans are taken before exercise and at various times during exercise. If part of the ventricular wall doesn't function as well during exercise as it does at rest, it probably does not have a good blood supply, and coronary artery disease may be present.

Another type of nuclear medicine scan is used to assess the coronary arteries and the circulation of the heart specifically. This is properly called a coronary perfusion (circulation to the heart muscle) scan, but it is more commonly called a thallium scan, after the name of the nuclear medication used in this test. Unlike technetium, thallium does not bind to red blood cells. It specifically enters the muscle cells of the heart after it has been carried there by the coronary arteries.

In a perfusion scan, the scanning cameras detect the amount of thallium taken up by the heart muscle. If an area of the muscle has poor circulation, it will take up the thallium much more slowly than the surrounding muscle. On the scan this area will appear lighter than the surrounding heart muscle. If there is an area of scar tissue from a previous heart attack, it will not take up the thallium at all. The perfusion scan may also be done during and after exercise.

The last type of nuclear medicine scan used to diagnose heart problems is a ventilation perfusion scan of the lungs. This test involves using two types of radioactive tracers. The first is the ventilation scan. The radioactive tracer is contained in an inert gas, usually xenon, which the patient breathes in. The pictures taken after this show the lungs, or at least the portion of the lungs that can exchange gas.

The second portion is a perfusion scan. This involves injecting a radioactive tracer in the blood. This tracer is taken up by the lungs as the blood flows through them. By comparing the ventilation scan to the perfusion scan, doctors can determine whether the blood flow to part of the lung is blocked. This scan usually is performed in people who are suspected of having pulmonary embolism, blood clots in a vein that have moved to the lungs.

The nuclear medicine scans give more accurate information regarding the heart's function and coronary artery disease than does an exercise EKG, but the scans are more complex and expensive than the EKG. The risks are also slightly higher. As with an exercise EKG, it is possible for a person to have a heart attack during the exercise portion of the test, although this is very rare. A very few people have an allergic reaction to the medication used in the test. In extremely rare cases, such a reaction can be life-threatening, but the doctors performing the test are always immediately ready to treat such a reaction.

The amount of radiation exposure during a nuclear medicine test is minimal—about the same as you would receive during a series of abdominal X rays. The technicians often wear special radiation equipment, such as lead-lined gloves or aprons, which may seem to suggest that a lot of radiation is present. Actually, this is required only because they are exposed to the radiation all day long for many years. The one-time exposure the patient receives is minimal.

Even nuclear medicine tests do not give all the information a cardiologist may need. They do not actually show the coronary arteries or heart valves, for example. In order to visualize the heart more directly, an echocardiography or a cardiac catheterization may be needed.

Echocardiography (Ultrasound Examination of the Heart)

Echocardiography is similar in principle and practice to the ultrasound examination that most pregnant women undergo. It is a very simple, totally noninvasive test used to evaluate the heart's structure.

The test uses a machine that sends very high frequency sound waves through the chest wall. Some of the sound waves bounce back toward the transducer each time they pass through any object in their path. By analyzing the echoes from the sound waves, a computer can tell the shape, density, and distance from the transducer of the different organs.

Several varieties of echocardiography each give slightly different information. The most common type is 2-D (for two-dimensional) echocardiography, which shows an actual cross section of the heart. This can be used to evaluate the size of the ventricles, the structure of the valves, and the contracting ability of the heart muscle. A 2-D examination may also be used to evaluate the abdominal aorta or carotid arteries (the large arteries in the neck that supply the brain) to check for atherosclerosis plaques or aneurysms.

M-mode echocardiography doesn't show the structure of the heart like 2-D does, but it provides accurate measurements of the heart valves and their openings. It is therefore the most important form of echocardiography for persons with valvular disease. This evaluation may be performed every year to see whether valvular disease is worsening. It may also be used to check for thrombosis (blood clots) in the heart or blood vessels.

Doppler echocardiography and Color Doppler echocardiography provide a picture similar to 2-D echocardiography, but in addition measure the speed and direction of blood flow. They are especially useful for determining the degree of backward flow from leaky valves. Most 2-D echocardiography machines now include Doppler capabilities. Doppler echocardiography also provides a way to measure the pressures in the pulmonary artery, an evaluation that used to require a very invasive test.

No risk is involved in an echocardiogram. Whichever type of echocardiography is used, the examination itself is very simple. You simply lie still while a technician moves the transducer over your chest, obtaining the different views needed for the examination. The sound waves cannot be felt, and there is no discomfort during the examination. Although performed infrequently, exercise echocardiography may be used. The exercise portion of the test is similar to that used for a stress EKG or MUGA scan.

Very rarely, transesophageal echocardiography must be used to visualize some portion of the heart that is not visible through the chest wall. This involves swallowing a cord containing an ultrasound transducer so that it is in the esophagus behind the heart. While it sounds awful, the procedure is performed after the throat is numbed and usually with intravenous sedation. Most people who undergo transesophageal echocardiography do not find it particularly unpleasant.

Computed Tomography (CT) Scans and Magnetic Resonance Imaging (MRI)

Computed tomography is a specialized type of X ray. Rather than just shooting a beam of X rays through the body in one direction, a CT scanner sends multiple beams through the body in many directions. The machine uses a sophisticated computer to reassemble the information into a two-dimensional cross-sectional picture that provides clear details.

CT scans involve lying on a stretcher that is passed through a large circular opening that contains the scanning equipment. It causes no discomfort, but the scan involves lying still for fifteen to thirty minutes until all the images have been obtained. Occasionally, X-ray contrast dye may be injected through an intravenous line to enhance the quality of the scan.

CT scans are not dangerous, although they do expose you to a little more radiation than standard X rays do. The amount is not even close to what is considered a harmful dose, however. As with any medication, an allergic reaction to the contrast dye is possible, but otherwise the procedure carries no risk of complications.

Magnetic resonance scans are very similar to CT scans, but they use a very high strength magnetic field rather than X rays. An MRI scanner is usually a tunnel-shaped device rather than the large circle of a CT scanner. A few people feel claustrophobic in an MRI scanner.

Neither test is used frequently for heart patients, though they may be useful to look for blood clots or problems in the sac surrounding the heart. They also can be used to check the lungs for a variety of heart-related conditions.

Invasive Tests of the Heart and Blood Vessels

Most invasive tests of the heart seem very similar to the patient. Usually they are done in the same location in the hospital, called the cardiac catheterization lab or the angiography suite. A single test or several tests and treatments may be done at one time. All these tests start with cardiac catheterization, the placement of long thin tubes (catheters) into the various chambers of the heart.

The invasive tests are needed because they most accurately define the patient's heart disease. They are never first-line tests, however, because they are invasive. There is always a small risk involved in an invasive test that is not present in a noninvasive examination. They are also very expensive. For these reasons, patients do not undergo invasive tests until doctors are fairly certain that some degree of heart disease is present.

Cardiac Catheterization

All invasive tests begin with cardiac catheterization. It is a minor surgical procedure, and preparation for cardiac catheterization is the same as preparation for surgery. The night before, you are asked to shower with antibiotic soap. You may need to shave your groin area or the inside of your elbows. Usually you should have nothing to eat or drink after midnight (although you should take any prescribed medicine on

schedule with a small sip of water), and you may be given a mild sedative to help you sleep.

The catheterization is done in a specialized room that combines the
equipment of an operating room with a large number of specialized
X-ray machines. The personnel in the room are scrubbed and dressed in
surgical gowns. Before the procedure is begun, an intravenous line will
be started in one of your arms, and you will receive some sedation and
medicine for pain. Although you need to remain awake during the
catheterization so that you can cooperate with the cardiologist, most
people don't remember the procedure very well.

Before the procedure begins, the area that the catheter will be introduced through is scrubbed and painted with an iodine solution, and the
rest of your body is covered in sterile drapes. EKG leads will be applied
to your chest and back, an automated blood pressure cuff to one arm,
and an oxygen sensor slipped over one finger. Usually you will receive
some supplemental oxygen by a mask.

To begin the procedure, the skin over the blood vessel chosen to receive the catheter (usually the femoral artery in the groin) will be
numbed by a local anesthetic. A tube called a sheath, which is about ¼
inch in diameter, is inserted into a blood vessel. The cardiologist can
then insert and remove several different catheters through the sheath
without having to stick any more needles into the blood vessel. You may
feel some tugging as the different catheters are placed in the sheath, but
there should be no more pain after that point.

If the arteries in the groin are not appropriate for the catheterization
(for instance, there may be atherosclerosis of these arteries), then the
artery above your elbow may be used. In this case, a small incision may
be made for insertion of the sheath, but otherwise the procedure is no
different than if the groin is used.

Once the sheath has been properly placed in the blood vessel, a
variety of catheters can be placed to inject dye for special X rays, mea-

sure pressures in various blood vessels and in the chambers of the heart, or perform other tests. After the tests are over the sheath may be removed, or it may be left in place for twenty-four hours or so in case other tests are needed. One or two stitches may be needed to close the puncture wound from the sheath, or a small dressing may be all that is needed.

One of the technicians will hold manual pressure over the puncture site for about fifteen minutes after the sheath is removed, to make sure that no bleeding occurs. Even so, a small amount of bruising and bleeding is expected. If a large swelling occurs around the puncture site, bleeding into the tissues is probably the cause. If this occurs, it may be necessary to make a small incision to repair the blood vessel and remove the old blood.

Following the procedure, you will be taken to a recovery room for an hour or so. Usually you will not be allowed to walk (or move your arm if that site was used) for about six hours after the procedure. It is usually recommended that you drink a lot of liquid to help flush the dye from your system.

Complications of the sheath insertion and removal are rare, though infection can occur. In a very few cases, the site of sheath insertion can form an aneurysm in the artery. In a few other cases, the process of sheath insertion damages the inside of the blood vessel itself, which must be repaired. Since nerves are located next to arteries, it is possible for a nerve to be irritated during the procedure. The symptoms of this are a radiating pain down the limb the procedure was performed in. It usually resolves in a few weeks. Overall, fewer than 1 out of 100 persons have such complications, however.

Coronary Angiography

One of the most common reasons to perform a cardiac catheterization is for coronary angiography. In this test a catheter is inserted through the sheath and threaded up the aorta to the area where the coronary arteries begin (see Figures 1-1 and 9-1). While an X-ray machine visualizes the catheter tip, the cardiologist will use various curved guide wires to advance it until it enters one of the coronary arteries.

Radiopaque dye (a dye that blocks X rays) is then injected through the catheter while a rapid series of X rays is taken. The dye fills the coronary artery, and the X rays will show any areas of narrowing that have occurred from coronary artery disease. These pictures show the exact extent and severity of coronary artery disease and allow the doctors to determine how best to treat it.

During the angiogram, it is not unusual for your heart to skip a beat, or to have a brief episode of very rapid beats. This is not cause for concern, and one of the technicians in the suite is always monitoring your EKG to make sure none of the beats are dangerous and to administer medications if needed. In addition to abnormal beats, the injection of dye sometimes makes people feel warm or flushed, and very occasionally makes them nauseated for a few minutes. These symptoms will pass in a short time.

During the procedure the cardiologist may roll the table you are on in one direction or another to get proper views for the X-ray cameras. He may also ask you to hold a deep breath or to cough. If you have symptoms of chest pain or light-headedness, you should tell the cardiologist at once.

The complications of angiography include those that can occur from the sheath insertion. It is also possible for the angiography procedure to irritate the heart, causing irregular beats for a few hours. If this occurs, the cardiologist may want to monitor your heartbeat in the hospital overnight. A rare complication is allergy to the dye injected for angiography. This is occasionally severe, but can generally be treated with drugs.

Since angiography is performed on persons with coronary artery disease, it is possible for the stress of the procedure to cause a heart attack. The cardiologist has several methods, including "clot-busting" drugs and angioplasty (see below), to treat such a heart attack before any permanent damage is done. Severe rhythm irregularities or cardiac arrest can also occur and require resuscitation. Finally, the catheters themselves may cause damage to the aorta, coronary arteries, or the heart. The risk of such severe complications is low (about 1 in 1,000), but your cardiologist should still discuss them with you before the procedure.

Left Heart Catheterization and Ventriculography

Ventriculography (injecting dye into the left ventricle and taking X rays) is often performed at the same time as angiography, but it may also be performed without angiography for people with heart disease other than coronary artery disease. The procedure is almost the same as for angiography, but the catheter is placed into the left ventricle rather than the coronary arteries.

Ventriculography allows a very accurate assessment of the pumping abilities of the left ventricle as well as evaluation of the function of the valves. It may also be used in some cases of congenital heart defects to see if there is a leak between the various chambers of the heart. The complications and recovery following ventriculography are similar to those of angiography, but there is less likelihood of heart attack or irregular heartbeat.

Arteriography (Angiogram)

An arteriogram, or angiogram, is very similar to ventriculography, but instead of visualizing the heart, dye is used to visualize the interior of one or more arteries. The procedure is generally used to evaluate atherosclerosis or aneurysms of the aorta or carotid arteries. The risks, recovery, and complications are similar to those of ventriculography.

Right Heart Catheterization

All the above tests involve inserting catheters through an artery toward the left side of the heart—all the way to the left ventricle in the case of ventriculography. In some cases it is important to evaluate the right side of the heart. In this case, a catheter is inserted through a vein and then threaded to the right side of the heart. Since this type of heart catheterization does not require an artery to be punctured, it does not always require all the specialized equipment that left heart catheterization does.

Right heart catheterization also requires insertion of a sheath, while it is inserted into a large central vein rather than an artery. The femoral vein in the groin and the subclavian vein under the collarbone are most commonly used for this purpose. Sterile technique is used, but the procedure may be carried out in a normal hospital bed.

Because the pressure in veins is much lower than that in arteries, there is much less risk of bleeding or aneurysm formation after insertion of a central venous sheath. When the subclavian vein under the collarbone is used for sheath insertion, there is about a 1 percent chance of the needle nicking the lung, which may result in a collapsed lung. A partially collapsed lung may recover on its own, but sometimes a tube must be inserted into the chest between two ribs to reexpand a collapsed lung. Despite this complication, the subclavian vein is often preferred because threading a catheter to the heart from this vein is far easier than trying to reach it from any other vein.

Inserting a central venous sheath provides doctors with information about the pressures in the veins at the point where they enter the heart. This information can help decide what type of medication is needed to treat a heart attack or other cardiac condition. It is not unusual for a sheath to remain in place for several days to help guide the treatment and monitor the patient's response following a heart attack or other heart problem. Once inserted, the catheter is no more uncomfortable than any other type of intravenous line.

Pulmonary Artery Catheterization

Frequently a catheter is inserted through the central venous sheath and fed through the right ventricle into the pulmonary artery. This type of catheter is often called a Swan-Ganz catheter, after the gentlemen who developed it. Pulmonary artery catheters can also be left in place for several days to provide information about the heart's function during critical illness.

The standard pulmonary artery catheter has multiple openings along its length and may also have an infrared sensor at its tip. With each heartbeat the catheter tells physicians the pressure in the central veins, the right ventricle, and the pulmonary artery. If it has an infrared sensor, it also measures the oxygen concentration of the blood returning to the heart. With a bedside computer attached, the pulmonary artery catheter can determine what the cardiac output is—the volume of blood the heart is pumping each minute. Finally, an electrical pacemaker can be inserted through the catheter, should that become necessary.

Obviously, the pulmonary artery catheter can be of vital importance in a critically ill person with heart disease. In most cases it is left in place for two or three days until the patient stabilizes. The catheter is not entirely without risk, however. Inserting it through the heart into the pulmonary artery can cause abnormal heart rhythms. Very rarely, the catheter can cause damage to the heart or the pulmonary artery.

Electrophysiology

In some people with severe abnormal heart rhythms, the EKG does not provide enough information to determine what is causing the abnormality. In a few other cases it is necessary to determine exactly where the abnormality is so that it can be surgically corrected. In these cases it may be necessary to perform invasive cardiac electrophysiology studies—studies of the electrical function of the heart.

These studies are performed just like heart catheterization (usually through the right side of the heart, but occasionally through the left side). The catheter inserted has several microelectrodes near its tip. These are connected to a specialized EKG machine that records the activity from each electrode. As the catheter is inserted, it is visualized on an X ray while the electrical activity of the heart at its tip is monitored. By determining the location of the catheter when its electrodes sense the abnormal activity, it is possible to tell exactly what part of the heart or conducting system is affected.

Electrophysiology studies are often very lengthy, both because it can take quite a while to find the proper location and because various medications to treat the dysrhythmia may be tried during the study. It is not unusual for these studies to last three to five hours, not including time in the recovery room.

The risks of electrophysiologic studies are similar to those for right heart catheterization, but there is a much higher risk of an abnormal rhythm occurring during the study. This is in part because the catheter must be placed near the abnormal part of the heart, where it can cause irritation, but most of the risk is because persons requiring the study are much more likely than other heart patients to have severe arrhythmias.

Chapter 8

MEDICATIONS USED TO TREAT HEART PROBLEMS

Almost every person with significant heart disease takes medication, often several different ones. Some people just "take what the doctor prescribes" without understanding what the medicine is doing and what side effects it may have. With dozens of companies marketing several medications each, it is more important now than at any time in the past for you to become familiar with the medications you are taking.

Prescribing medications for heart disease remains an art as much as a science. Doctors know what effect they are trying to get with a certain medication, but they can never be absolutely certain that a given medicine will work in a particular case. Let's say, for example, the doctor wants to slow your heart rate. The class of drugs known as beta blockers is good for this, so one of them may be prescribed. At last count, there were twenty-three different beta blockers (including all the manufacturers' brands) to choose from.

If any one of these were clearly better for all patients, there wouldn't be twenty-three choices on the market. Each medication has a slightly different "side effect profile"; that is, it is more likely to cause some side effects and less likely to cause others. The doctor will prescribe one that he or she thinks will be well tolerated by you and ask you to try it for a few weeks. If it is not effective, or causes unpleasant side effects, the doctor will try another medication. The doctor knows that it may take two or three trials to find the best medication for you, though many physicians fail to explain this clearly.

Since each person responds slightly differently to each medication, the doctor will reexamine you to see if the medication has had the desired effect. The physician also will listen to your reports about changes in symptoms and the occurrence of any side effects, and then determine if a change is necessary.

If you are aware of what the medication is supposed to accomplish, why it has been prescribed, and what the potential side effects are, you will be able to give the doctor a clear report. If you notice a side effect from the medication, call the doctor rather than waiting until your next scheduled appointment. Your doctor may go ahead and change the medication to one you might tolerate better.

General Information About Medications

Names

Confusion about medication usually begins with names. Sometimes the same medication is marketed under several names, making it difficult to know exactly what you are taking. Every medication has at least two names: a generic (or chemical) name and a trade name assigned by a specific manufacturer. When a drug is first developed and released, the original manufacturer has exclusive rights to produce that drug for several years. During this time only the trade-name drug is available, though it may sometimes be referred to by its generic name.

After the exclusive period is over, any manufacturer can make and market the drug. A generic drug manufacturer may produce the drug and sell it to pharmacists under its generic name. Additionally, another company may produce the same drug and market it under a different trade name.

For example, verapamil is the generic name of a common heart medication. For several years verapamil was only marketed by the company that developed it under the trade name Calan. Once its patent ran out, the original company continued to market the drug as Calan, but it also became available as a generic drug and was marketed by other companies under the trade names Isoptin and Verelan. All these drugs are the same chemical. Assuming the quality control at the various companies is equal, all will have exactly the same effect and can be freely substituted for each other.

Additionally, groups of related medications are classified according to the overall effect they have on the body, and the specific effect they have on chemicals in the cells of the body. Each drug belongs to a specific group. To use the above example, verapamil was the first (and for a while the only) calcium channel blocker. There are now a dozen other calcium channel blockers, each with its own generic name and at least one trade name. These other calcium channel blockers are chemically different from verapamil and have slightly different effects and side effects.

Doses

Dosage of medication refers to the amount you take. The dose is usually noted as the weight of medication contained in the tablet, measured in milligrams (mg). Each medication has its own dosage range, which is the amount usually required to create an effect. For a given medication, some people will benefit at a much lower dose than others. One drug may have a dosage range of 10 to 20 mg a day, while another may have a range of 250 to 500 mg a day. This doesn't mean the first drug is more powerful than the second. Both are expected to have a similar effect as long as the proper dose is administered.

Drugs also have a dosage interval, meaning how often you must take it. The dosage interval depends on how long the drug remains in your body. The body gets rid of some chemicals very rapidly, while others remain a fairly long time. Many drugs are available as long-acting or slowly absorbed preparations that can be taken less frequently. These drugs usually have a two-letter abbreviation after their name, such as LA (long-acting), CR (controlled release), or SR (sustained release).

Whatever the dosage interval, it is important that you space the medication out so your body has a fairly constant level. If a medication is prescribed three times a day, the pills should be taken about eight hours apart. If you take one early in the morning, another after dinner, and the third at bedtime, you will actually have very little drug in your system during the afternoon and too much at night.

Side Effects

Every medication will cause some side effects, although ideally these are not very noticeable. Each medication is tested before it becomes available to the public to determine its side effect profile, a list of the most frequently noted side effects. Your doctor will take the side effect profile into account when prescribing medications for you. For example, if you have trouble with nausea, the doctor will try to pick a medication that is less likely to cause nausea. Remember, however, the profile cannot guarantee that certain side effects won't occur. It simply states that they are less likely.

In many cases, side effects are temporary. If the medication is particularly important for your condition, your doctor may ask you to bear with side effects for a week or two in the hope that they will go away. Many medications, for example, will cause you to feel tired or weak the first few days that you take them. If a side effect is severe, however, the medication should generally be stopped and another substituted.

Indications

Each medicine has a particular indication, a condition that the medication should benefit. Some medications have several indications and may therefore be used for any of several reasons. Verapamil, for example, lowers blood pressure, prevents certain types of dysrhythmia, and may prevent angina. People with very different types of heart disease may benefit from verapamil.

In a similar manner, medications from several classifications can have similar effects on the body. High blood pressure may be lowered with diuretic medications, calcium channel blockers, beta blockers, and several other types of medication. The choice of which class to use for each indication depends on a lot of factors, especially the presence of other diseases.

Your doctor will monitor you to determine how effective the medication is for your particular indication. Just as side effects vary from patient to patient, the effectiveness will also vary. Some people will not experience any change in blood pressure with verapamil, while others will have a dramatic result. Usually, if a medication is ineffective, the doctor will try another one in the same classification. If two or three medicines in the class are ineffective, then it may be beneficial to try another class of medications.

The Commonly Used Medications by Groups

Medications are grouped into several categories based on the specific effects they have in the body. Medications in the same group tend to have similar effects, side effects, and indications. For this reason, we will discuss the general groups of medications together. Your pharmacist will usually give you a fact sheet that will tell you which class of drug the medicine belongs in, and will usually give you more details about the specific drug. If the fact sheet doesn't list drug classification, or you're not sure which group the medication you're taking belongs in, you can look it up in appendices C and D.

Nitrates

Actions and Indications

The nitrates are a class of drugs that have been used frequently by heart patients for over seventy-five years. The drugs in this class work by dilating (enlarging) blood vessels. Dilating arteries has the effect of lowering blood pressure and decreasing the workload of the heart. Dilating the veins allows blood to pool in the legs and abdomen, further decreasing the workload of the heart. These drugs may or may not dilate the coronary arteries. Their effectiveness is based more on their ability to lower the heart's workload than on their effect on the coronary arteries.

The primary indication for nitrates is to prevent or stop angina. Since angina occurs when the heart is working so hard that it can't get enough blood flow, the nitrates, which reduce the heart's workload in two ways, should effectively stop most angina attacks. In the past, nitrates were also used to treat hypertension, but they have been largely replaced by other drugs for this purpose.

Commonly Used Nitrates

By far the most commonly used medication in the nitrate class of drugs is nitroglycerin. This drug is supplied in many different forms: tablets, capsules, ointment, skin patches, and even a throat spray. Generally, the drug is supplied and used in two ways: long-acting preparations that prevent angina attacks and rapid-onset preparations that treat an attack once it begins.

Rapidly acting forms of nitroglycerin must be dissolved under the tongue. Veins under the tongue immediately carry the medication throughout the body. When medication is absorbed through the stomach, it passes through the liver, which removes a large portion of the drug before it ever gets to the circulatory system. Tablets that dissolve under the tongue (such as Nitrostat) are the rapidly acting form of nitroglycerin most frequently used, but an oral spray (Nitrolingual Spray) is also used.

Long-acting forms of nitroglycerin include capsules (Nitro-Bid) that are taken like any other medicine and tablets (Nitrogard) that are dissolved between the cheek and gum. Since nitroglycerin is steadily absorbed through the skin, an ointment form (Nitrol) can achieve the same effect. It can also be administered through slow-release skin patches (Nitro-Dur, Nitro-Disc, and others).

Three other medications are often used instead of long-acting nitroglycerin: isosorbide dinitrate (Isordil, Sorbitrate, Dilatrate); pentaerythrityl tetranitrate (whose manufacturer wisely shortened the trade name to Peritrate); and erythrityl tetranitrate (Cardilate). All these medications are pills taken on a regular schedule to prevent angina. None starts working fast enough to stop angina attacks that have already begun. Although their action is almost identical to nitroglycerin, some people have fewer side effects with these medications.

Precautions and Side Effects

Most of the side effects caused by the nitrates are related to the dilation of blood vessels. Most people experience side effects when they first take these drugs, but they usually wear off in a few days. Side effects are more likely, and may be more severe, with the rapidly acting nitroglycerin preparations.

Dizziness and light-headedness may occur because the blood pressure is lowered. Lying down or elevating the legs will usually relieve these symptoms. A few people actually faint if they stand up rapidly after taking nitroglycerin. For this reason, it is important that you stand slowly and make certain you don't feel faint before you start walking. For the same reason, you shouldn't drive or operate dangerous equipment for the first few days after you start taking nitrates.

Because these medications also dilate the blood vessels in the head, some people get a throbbing headache after taking nitroglycerin. This headache may be relieved by sitting upright and is usually stopped by Tylenol or another analgesic. The headache will generally disappear within an hour after taking a rapidly acting nitroglycerin preparation. If you get headaches from a long-acting form, they should stop three to five days after starting the medication. If headache persists, your doctor may need to substitute a different nitrate medication.

People develop some tolerance to all the nitrate drugs. This means that over time, the drugs don't work quite as effectively as they did at first. Because of tolerance, your doctor may increase the dose after a few weeks or months. Whenever your dose is increased, you may reexperience any side effects you had when you first started the medication, although they are usually less severe.

Once you have taken long-acting nitrates for any length of time, you should never stop them suddenly. Stopping nitrates suddenly can cause rebound, a sudden worsening of angina or high blood pressure. When it is time to stop this medication, your doctor will have you taper it off safely.

In case you were wondering (a few people do), the nitroglycerin used in heart medications is the same chemical used as an explosive. Because only tiny amounts are needed for the medicinal effect, there is no danger of your pills exploding.

Interactions with Other Drugs

The major concern for people taking nitrates is that they can interact with other medications that also dilate the blood vessels. Alcohol is a potent vasodilator, so you should be very cautious about taking nitrates and drinking alcohol. Many people taking nitrates experience dizziness or headache if they have even one alcoholic drink.

Other medications that reduce blood pressure, such as antihypertensives, beta blockers, and calcium channel blockers, can also interact with nitrates to cause blood pressure drop. This does not mean these medications should never be combined; many people take several of these medications in combination. It does mean that you must be watched carefully for the first few days when you start a new medicine from one of these groups. As always, be certain your doctor is aware of all the medications you are already taking whenever a new medication is prescribed for you.

Beta Blockers

Available since the 1970s, beta blockers have become one of the most widely used heart medications. This is reflected by the number of drugs of this class on the market. At last count thirteen different beta-blocking drugs were available in the United States, and another half dozen used in Europe. Each has at least one trade-name preparation available, and most are available in a generic form.

Actions and Indications

The beta blockers work by blocking certain actions of the sympathetic nervous system. As a result of this blocking, they reduce heart rate, lower blood pressure, and reduce the contracting strength of the heart. The net result of all three effects is that the heart does not work nearly as hard and therefore requires less oxygen and blood flow. Beta blockers may also stop certain kinds of dysrhythmias.

The beta blockers are most commonly prescribed for people with coronary artery disease. By decreasing the workload on the heart, they decrease the frequency and severity of angina attacks. They are often used along with nitrates for this reason, especially for people who tend to have angina during exertion. There is also some evidence that taking beta blockers after a first heart attack may slightly reduce the risk of a second attack. Beta blockers are also used to treat some types of rapid heartbeat and a few other kinds of dysrhythmia.

Beta blockers are also used to treat hypertension, especially in people under forty years of age. Although they are usually not the first drug chosen for hypertension, they are especially suitable for people with high blood pressure and coronary artery disease. Because many people do have both hypertension and coronary disease, there are several combination medications containing both a beta blocker and a diuretic (medication to remove fluid). These combination medications may also be used for people who need a beta blocker but also have mild congestive heart failure.

Commonly Used Beta Blockers

The first beta blocker released was propranolol (Inderal), which remains commonly used today. It is also available as a long-acting preparation (Inderal LA) that only needs to be taken twice a day. Nadolol (Corgard) and timolol (Blocadren) are very similar to propranolol but have a longer duration of action. They can often be taken just once a day.

Metoprolol (Lopressor) and atenolol (Tenormin) have similar effects on the heart but have fewer effects on other organs. They are therefore known as cardioselective beta blockers. These drugs are often used in people with lung disease or diabetes, since nonselective beta blockers may cause problems for people with these conditions. Selective beta blockers may not be as effective as the other drugs for treating hypertension, however.

Pindolol (Visken), a nonselective beta blocker, and acebutolol (Sectral), a cardioselective beta blocker, are less likely than the other beta blockers to cause slow heart rates. They are sometimes used for people who are predisposed to bradycardia (very slow heart rates). Nadolol and atenolol seem to have fewer side effects on the central nervous system than the other beta blockers and may sometimes be used for people who become drowsy or confused when taking beta blockers.

Most of the above medications are available in preparations combining them with a diuretic. Inderide and Inderide LA combine propranolol and hydrochlorothiazide (a widely used diuretic). Lopressor HCT, Corzide, Tenoretic, and Viskazide are similar combinations of hydrochlorothiazide with metoprolol, nadolol, atenolol, and pindolol, respectively.

Labetalol (Trandate, Normodyne) is not only a beta blocker but also blocks alpha receptors, another part of the sympathetic nervous system. The overall effect of this medication is lowered blood pressure without much change in heart rate or the contracting ability of the heart. It is sometimes used instead of beta blockers for persons with congestive heart failure and coronary artery disease. It does have a higher rate of side effects than the pure beta-blocking medications. Labetalol is also combined with hydrochlorothiazide as the medication Normozide.

Precautions and Side Effects

The most significant side effects of beta blockers occur in people who have heart failure, diabetes, or lung problems. Beta blockers, especially the nonselective ones, can cause the bronchial tubes of people with lung disease to constrict, resulting in wheezing and shortness of breath. They can also lower the blood sugar in people with diabetes and mask the symptoms that usually occur with low blood sugar. Combination beta blockers and diuretics are especially likely to cause trouble for diabetic patients. Metoprolol and atenolol are least likely to cause problems for diabetic patients.

All beta blockers, whether cardioselective or not, can worsen the symptoms of heart failure. The symptoms of worsening heart failure may include shortness of breath, an inability to lie flat without becoming short of breath, and increased swelling. If any of the above symptoms occur, you should contact your doctor immediately.

Less significant side effects occur in some people during the first weeks of taking beta blockers. These include dizziness or even fainting, weakness, vomiting, trouble sleeping, and depression. If you experience any of these symptoms you should let your doctor know, but do not stop taking the medication until the doctor directs you to do so. Less frequent side effects include sexual difficulties (in males, especially), headache, confusion, loss of appetite, and allergic reactions (a rash or hives). These side effects are more likely to occur in people over sixty years of age. Atenolol, nadolol, and metoprolol are less likely to cause central nervous system effects like confusion and insomnia.

Persons taking beta blockers should not drive or operate equipment until they have taken the medication for several days and are comfortable with it. They should also be careful about working in high places or standing up suddenly. During hot weather, persons taking these medications should make sure they take in plenty of fluids, since they cannot tolerate dehydration well. They also should avoid exposure to strong sunlight, since these drugs may intensify sunburn.

Interactions with Other Drugs

Like the nitrates, beta blockers may cause people to have significant blood pressure drops if they drink alcohol. Beta blockers also increase the sedating effects of antihistamines. As mentioned earlier, beta blockers can alter the response of blood sugar in diabetics, so diabetic patients may need to adjust their medications or food intake. Beta blockers also can interact with certain antidepressant medications. If you are taking antidepressants and beta blockers, make sure your doctor is aware of this.

Calcium Channel Blockers

Calcium channel blockers became available in the 1980s and have become widely prescribed for a variety of heart conditions. This class of drugs is being actively researched by the pharmaceutical industry. New calcium channel blockers become available almost every year.

Actions and Indications

The calcium channel blockers work by interfering with calcium flow in the muscles of the heart and blood vessels. Even though they work in areas of the body that are entirely different from the areas where beta blockers work, the overall results of taking calcium channel blockers are similar to those obtained with beta blockers. Calcium channel blockers reduce heart rate, lower blood pressure, and reduce the contracting strength of the heart. They may also dilate the coronary arteries and stop certain kinds of dysrhythmias.

Unlike the beta blockers, which all have the same general effects, different calcium channel blockers vary quite a bit in their predominant effects. Some dramatically lower the blood pressure without affecting heart rate very much. Others slow the heart rate and decrease the contracting ability of the heart quite a bit.

Not surprisingly, calcium blockers are often prescribed for indications similar to those the beta blockers are used for: to lower blood pressure, decrease the number of angina attacks, and to treat certain dysrhythmias. Calcium channel blockers are most often prescribed to prevent angina, because of their ability to increase blood flow to the heart while decreasing the amount of work the heart does. They are especially indicated for people who have angina at unexpected times rather than just during exertion.

Calcium channel blockers can also be used to treat hypertension. They are frequently substituted for beta blockers in people who have lung disease or diabetes, since calcium channel blockers do not affect the bronchial tubes or blood sugar. In a few cases, they are used in addition to beta blockers, but this must be done cautiously, since the side effects of these two medications tend to add to each other.

Some recent studies have suggested that certain calcium channel blockers can also be useful for patients with congestive heart failure. Other studies indicate that they should be avoided in persons with this condition. Currently, they are not a first-line treatment for congestive heart failure, and when they are used, patients should be monitored carefully.

Commonly Used Calcium Channel Blockers

Verapamil (Calan, Isoptin, Verelan) was the first calcium channel blocker introduced. Of all the calcium channel blockers, verapamil has the most profound effects on the heart itself, slowing the pulse, decreasing the heart's contraction strength, and stopping some forms of dysrhythmia. It does lower blood pressure but does not dilate the blood vessels as much as some other drugs in this class.

Nifedipine (Procardia, Adalat) has fewer effects on the heart but profoundly dilates the arteries throughout the body. It is frequently used to treat hypertension, especially in severe cases. It has a short dosage interval, so it must be taken more frequently than many of the other medications in this class. Diltiazem (Cardizem) has effects somewhat between those of nifedipine and verapamil. Nicardipine (Cardene), is-radipine (DynaCirc), and felodipine (Plendil) are all similar medications to diltiazem, affecting both the heart and the blood vessels.

Precautions and Side Effects

Overall, this group of medications causes side effects less frequently than most cardiac drugs. When side effects do occur, they vary depending on the type of medication. Verapamil, and to a lesser extent the other drugs in this class, can cause a slow heart rate and worsen the symptoms of congestive heart failure. Nifedipine, and to a lesser extent the other drugs in this class, can cause dramatic drops in blood pressure, resulting in dizziness and even fainting. Any of these effects is an emergency, and your doctor (or a hospital if needed) should be called at once if you experience them.

Less severe side effects also occur but are rare. They may include nausea or constipation, difficulty urinating, and hair loss. A few people experience headache, trouble sleeping, and vivid dreams. As with beta blockers, side effects are more likely in people over sixty years of age. Persons taking calcium channel blockers should not drive or operate equipment until they have taken the medication for several days and are comfortable with it. They should also be careful about working in high places or standing up suddenly.

People with liver and kidney disease do not metabolize the calcium channel blocking drugs as quickly as other people. For this reason, they must take lower or less frequent doses.

Interactions with Other Drugs

Calcium channel blockers are quite likely to interact with other heart medications. People taking digitalis, antihypertensives, beta blockers, antidysrhythmic medications, and ACE inhibitors (see below) are likely to need to have the dose of these medications adjusted when they begin taking calcium channel blockers. This is especially true in the case of antihypertensives and beta blockers, since combining calcium channel blockers with these can cause extremely low blood pressure.

Antiseizure medications also can interact with calcium channel blockers, and the dose of these medications may need to be decreased. People taking medications for asthma or emphysema, especially the medication theophylline, should be monitored carefully. Calcium channel blockers may increase the amount of these medications in the bloodstream to dangerous levels.

The antacid medication cimetidine (Tagamet) should not be taken by people taking calcium channel blockers, since it can interfere with the metabolism of some of these drugs, resulting in an unintended overdose. Other antacid medications are safe.

Inotropes (Heart-Strengthening Medications)

A variety of inotropes are used intravenously in the hospital, but only the digitalis group are currently available for use as oral medications.

Actions and Indications

The inotropes cause weakened heart muscle cells to contract more vigorously. These drugs would not have an effect on a person with a normal heart, but they can cause dramatic improvement of heart function in people with heart failure. In most people with heart failure, taking inotropes reduces swelling and shortness of breath, improves exercise tolerance, and eliminates symptoms of orthopnea (shortness of breath when lying down).

The digitalis drugs also slow the conduction of beats through the electrical system of the heart. For this reason they are used to treat some forms of dysrhythmia.

Commonly Used Inotropes

Only two inotropic drugs are used frequently in the United States: digoxin (Lanoxin, Lanoxicaps) and digitoxin (Crystodigin). Digoxin has a longer dosing interval and only needs to be taken once a day. Otherwise, the two drugs are identical in their actions and very similar in their side effects.

Precautions and Side Effects

When taken by mouth, the amount of digitalis absorbed into the body varies quite a bit from person to person. For this reason, it is difficult for doctors to predict how much digitalis an individual will need. Generally, you will be started on a low dose of digoxin or digitoxin, and after a week or two the amount of medication in your blood will be measured. Based on the results of this measurement, the doctor will then alter the dose.

People often experience some mild side effects when they start taking digitalis preparations. These side effects, which include loss of appetite, drowsiness, and diarrhea, are generally mild and disappear in a few days. A few people experience more significant mental disturbance, including confusion, fainting, and even hallucinations. If these occur, you should stop the medication and talk to your doctor right away.

The digitalis drugs slow the heartbeat, and some people experience bradycardia (very slow pulse) when taking them. Other uncommon side effects include double vision, seeing a yellow-green halo around objects in bright light, decreased sex drive, and enlargement of the male breasts. Because of the possibility of visual disturbances, you should not drive for the first few days you take digitalis.

The most important precaution for people taking digitalis medications is to be aware that the difference between a therapeutic dose and an overdose is fairly small. If you have forgotten whether you took a day's pill or not, *do not take it*. Overdose symptoms can also result from interactions between digitalis drugs and other medications (see below). Symptoms of digitalis overdose include vision disturbances with halos, vomiting, irregular heartbeat, and confusion. If you develop such symptoms you should be transported (DO NOT DRIVE) to a hospital immediately.

Interactions with Other Drugs

Many drugs interfere with the body's ability to absorb the digitalis drugs. For this reason, people taking these drugs should not take any medications (even over-the-counter medicines) without consulting their doctor. Beta blockers, asthma medications, cortisone, and anti-seizure medication all raise the blood levels of digitalis. Cholesterol-reducing drugs, and even antacids and laxatives, can reduce the levels of digitalis.

Other drugs can interact with digitalis to cause an irregular heartbeat. Any cold pill that contains the medications ephedrine or pseudoephedrine can cause this effect, as can large amounts of caffeine or asthma medicine. Some antidepressant drugs can also interact with digitalis in this fashion.

Diuretics

Diuretic medications cause the body to get rid of water. There are several subcategories of diuretics, depending on what other substances leave the body along with water, and on the relative strength of the medication. Most diuretics cause the body to lose potassium. These types of diuretics are further separated into two groups: the thiazide diuretics (generally milder) and the loop diuretics (stronger). A third group, the potassium-sparing diuretics, tends to keep potassium in the body. All the medications in this group are considered mild diuretics.

Actions and Indications

Diuretics are used for two purposes. They are one of the first treatments selected (and often the only drug needed) for people with hypertension. They are also used to remove excess fluid from people who have swelling caused by congestive heart failure. Generally, thiazide diuretics are used for the treatment of hypertension and the more potent loop diuretics are used for the treatment of heart failure. People taking either of these medications may need to take potassium supplements or eat potassium-rich foods (bananas are a good source).

Potassium-sparing diuretics are used for people who have medical conditions that make potassium loss dangerous. More often, potassium-sparing diuretics are combined with a standard diuretic. Theoretically, this combination should balance out potassium loss, so that the person taking the combined medications does not have to take potassium supplements. Like most theories put into practice, this one works a lot of the time, but not always.

Commonly Used Diuretics

The most commonly prescribed thiazide diuretic is hydrochlorothiazide (Esidrix, HydroDiuril, Oretic). Other frequently used thiazides are chlorothiazide (Diuril) and methyclothiazide (Aquatensin, Enduron). Similar drugs include chlorthalidone (Hygroton, Thalitone) and metolazone (Zaroxolyn).

The potent loop diuretics are furosemide (Lasix), ethacrynic acid (Edecrin), and bumetanide (Bumex). Potassium-sparing diuretics include spironolactone (Aldactone), triamterene (Dyrenium), and amiloride (Midamor).

Combination diuretics generally combine hydrochlorothiazide and a potassium-sparing diuretic. Moduretic (hydrochlorothiazide and amiloride), Aldactazide (hydrochlorothiazide and spironolactone), and

Dyazide or Maxzide (hydrochlorothiazide and triamterene) are the most commonly used combination diuretics.

Precautions and Side Effects

All diuretics can disturb the body's balance of electrolytes, the small electrically charged chemicals such as potassium and sodium. Since almost every chemical function of the body requires a proper balance of electrolytes, these disturbances can cause significant problems. For this reason, blood chemistry studies are done before you begin these drugs and a week or two later.

Thiazide diuretics usually lower the potassium levels and may also lower sodium and calcium levels in the blood. Symptoms of low potassium include muscle cramps, dizziness, and a weak or irregular pulse. If you experience these symptoms, you should call your doctor right away. Your doctor may start you on potassium supplements when you start taking a thiazide diuretic, but this will depend on your initial blood chemistry results.

Some people also experience mood changes, headache, diarrhea, and thirst when starting thiazide diuretics. These symptoms usually go away in a few days. If not, another drug may be substituted. Thiazides can worsen sunburn or cause sun sensitivity in a few people. They also can raise the blood sugar, which can be a significant problem for diabetic patients, and they may cause a gout attack in people who are predisposed to this illness.

Loop diuretics are more likely to lower potassium than are the thiazide diuretics. Most people taking loop diuretics will need to take potassium supplements, and their blood potassium levels should be checked within a week of beginning the medication. People taking loop diuretics also become dehydrated easily and must be careful to drink plenty of fluid during hot weather. Symptoms of muscle cramps, weak or rapid pulse, and feeling faint when standing indicate a significant loss of potassium and fluid. If this occurs, you should contact your doctor immediately or be taken to a hospital.

Less frequent side effects of loop diuretics include ringing in the ears, unusual bleeding or bruising, jaundice (yellow color of the skin or eyes), and tingling or numbness in the hands and feet. You should stop the medication and call your doctor at once if any of these occur. Milder side effects may include stomach upset and sun sensitivity. Like the thiazides, loop diuretics may raise blood sugar levels and can trigger a gout attack.

The potassium-sparing diuretics are less likely to cause electrolyte abnormalities. They can, however, cause a few people to develop high potassium levels. This is more common in people who have kidney or liver disease, but it can occur in others as well. For this reason, people taking potassium-sparing diuretics should not use salt substitutes that contain potassium. Symptoms of high potassium levels include muscle weakness, confusion, and irregular heartbeat.

Spironolactone can occasionally cause heavy sweating, dizziness, menstrual irregularities, and change in sex drive. It may also cause excessive hair growth and voice changes in women, though these effects are quite rare. It may also cause sun sensitivity.

Triamterene may cause headache, weakness, anxiety, or confusion in a few people. It also has been reported to cause severe allergic reactions in rare cases. An unusual side effect of this drug is a rash or soreness in the mouth and throat. If this occurs, the medication will usually have to be changed, since this side effect worsens over time.

Interactions with Other Drugs

Any diuretic can have an additive effect with antihypertensive medications, causing a drop in blood pressure. Both thiazide and loop diuretics also interact with some antidepressants, causing a similar drop in blood pressure. Cortisone interacts with both the thiazide and the loop diuretics, worsening the potassium loss these drugs normally cause.

Persons taking lithium should not take any potassium-sparing diuretic, as this may cause lithium toxicity. Similarly, ACE inhibitors and potassium-sparing diuretics should not be taken together, since the combination can cause lethal increases in blood potassium levels. The potassium-sparing diuretics will reduce the blood levels of digitalis, so the dose of that medication may need to be adjusted after potassium-sparing diuretics are started.

Angiotensin Converting Enzyme (ACE) Inhibitors

The ACE inhibitors are a fairly recently developed class of drugs that offer a new method for treating certain types of heart disease. Like the calcium channel blockers, ACE inhibitors are being researched heavily by drug companies, and new medications in this class are introduced every year or two.

Actions and Indications

Angiotensin converting enzyme is a protein in the body that produces angiotensin II, a regulating chemical that increases the resistance of the arteries and raises the blood pressure. Angiotensin converting enzyme inhibitors slow this process, reducing the body's levels of angiotensin II. Decreasing angiotensin II levels lowers the blood pressure and reduces the amount of work the heart must do to pump blood.

The major uses of ACE inhibitors, therefore, are to treat hypertension and congestive heart failure. Although these drugs are used for patients with either problem, they are especially beneficial for those who have both congestive failure and hypertension. In such people, ACE inhibitors not only improve symptoms, they have been shown to slow the progression of heart failure and improve life expectancy.

These drugs have several advantages over other medications used for the same purposes. One advantage is that they preserve the blood flow to the kidneys, where other antihypertensive medications can decrease the kidneys' blood flow. ACE inhibitors also have a lower frequency of side effects than many other medications. Diabetic and renal failure patients, who often have side effects from blood pressure medications, are especially likely to benefit from ACE inhibitors.

ACE inhibitors are frequently used in combination with other medications that reduce the resistance of the arteries. The reason for this is simple: whenever an arterial dilating medication is given to a patient, the body increases its levels of angiotensin II to try to raise the blood pressure. By administering an ACE inhibiter, doctors can minimize this response, allowing lower doses of the first medication to be used.

Commonly Used ACE Inhibitors

The most commonly prescribed ACE inhibitors include captopril (Capoten), enalapril (Vasotec), lisinopril (Zestril, Prinivil), benazepril (Lotensin), and fosinopril (Monopril). These drugs are all similar in effectiveness, though one may be better for a given patient than another. They also have slightly different side effect profiles, though the differences are minimal compared to the variations between drugs in some other classes.

Precautions and Side Effects

ACE inhibitors are less likely to cause side effects than most other cardiac medications, but when side effects occur they may be severe. These drugs can cause the blood pressure to drop too far, resulting in dizziness or fainting. This is less frequent with ACE inhibitors than with most other antihypertensive medications, however. ACE inhibitors also cause nausea or a rash in a few people. They may also cause some people to retain too much potassium, so your doctor will probably check your potassium level a week or two after you start an ACE inhibitor.

In a very few patients (well less than 1 in 1,000), ACE inhibitors cause significant swelling of the lips and throat, a condition called angioedema. In a very few people, this can result in some obstruction of the airway and severe shortness of breath. If this occurs, you should go to an emergency room immediately. This complication can be easily treated, but could become life-threatening if ignored.

In extremely rare cases (less than 1 in 10,000), these drugs cause a severe drop in the white blood cell count. Since white blood cells fight infection, this condition can be very serious, even fatal. Your doctor will probably check your blood count every month or two after you've started these medications. If a drop in white blood cells is detected, it will reverse itself when the medication is discontinued.

Interactions with Other Drugs

When used with beta blockers, calcium channel blockers, or other antihypertensive medications, ACE inhibitors can cause a significant drop in blood pressure. A similar effect can occur in people who are taking diuretics, but this is usually temporary. Blood pressure drops may also occur if you drink alcohol while taking ACE inhibitors.

People taking ACE inhibitors should not take the antibiotic chloramphenicol, since this drug also can affect white blood cells. (Chloramphenicol is rarely used in any case.) They also should not take potassium or use salt substitutes containing potassium unless their doctor approves. Nonsteroidal anti-inflammatory drugs, such as ibuprofen (Motrin) or other arthritis medication, interferes with the action of

ACE inhibitors. Once you've started an ACE inhibitor, you should not take these drugs without your doctor's approval.

Other Antihypertension Medication

Most people with high blood pressure are treated with a diuretic. If the problem is severe, another medication is usually added. This may be a beta or calcium channel blocking drug or an ACE inhibitor. Many other drugs are used to treat hypertension that are not included in these categories, however. These antihypertensive drugs are loosely grouped into three categories: centrally acting drugs (those that work on the brain's blood pressure control centers), vasodilators (other than the nitrates), and drugs that affect the sympathetic nerves. This last group has largely been abandoned because of side effects, however.

Commonly Used Antihypertensives

Methyldopa (Aldomet, Aldoril, Aldoclor), clonidine (Catapres), and guanabenz (Wytensin) are all centrally acting drugs. These drugs have been used to treat hypertension for a long time but now are used less frequently than the beta blockers. All these drugs act by changing what the brain's blood pressure control centers consider "normal" and decreasing the signals the brain sends to the sympathetic nervous system.

Methyldopa, particularly, has fallen into disfavor because its side effects are unpleasant for many people. Clonidine and guanabenz seem to be better tolerated and are especially effective for people who have severe hypertension caused by kidney disease. Clonidine is also available as a skin patch medication, which only needs to be changed once a week.

The vasodilating drugs hydralazine (Apresoline) and minoxidil (Loniten) are generally used only in combination with other drugs. Because these drugs dilate the arteries, they reduce the workload of the heart. For this reason they are sometimes selected for people with congestive heart failure and hypertension. They are also used in patients who don't respond well to other drugs. Minoxidil, in particular, is effective in people with very high blood pressure.

Prazosin (Minipress) is the only drug affecting the sympathetic nerves that is still used frequently. It appears to be particularly effective in treating hypertension in young people and in people who have peripheral vascular disease. A few studies have also found that prazosin lowers triglyceride levels, making it a good choice for some people with hypertension and coronary artery disease.

Precautions and Side Effects

All these drugs cause a side effect known as postural hypotension, which means a drop in blood pressure that occurs when you change position. This is most likely when you move from a sitting to a standing position and usually is worse during the first few weeks of therapy. It is important to stand slowly, holding on to the edge of the chair in case you get dizzy. Once you have stood for a few seconds, you should be able to move about without trouble.

All these drugs are also associated with a phenomenon known as rebound hypertension. This means that if you stop taking them suddenly, your blood pressure will become higher than it was before you started the medication. Because of rebound hypertension, it is important that you never run out of this type of medication. Most people keep a three-day emergency supply on hand in case they forget to refill their prescription. If you find yourself without the medication while traveling, most pharmacists will give you a one- or two-day supply until you can get to a doctor's office.

Methyldopa has many side effects that limit the ability to tolerate it. Most people feel sedated and some feel depressed when taking this medication. It also causes sexual dysfunction or impotence in many men. Clonidine and guanabenz are less likely to cause side effects, though a few people report drowsiness, dry mouth, or sexual problems. Clonidine skin patches may cause itching in a small percentage of people.

Prazosin has also been reported to cause drowsiness and sexual dysfunction in men. Both prazosin and minoxidil may cause fluid retention, and minoxidil also can cause hair growth in usually hairless places. Most people do not experience these side effects, however, and the drowsiness usually lasts only a week or two.

Interactions with Other Drugs

Clonidine can interact with many antidepressants, especially fluoxetine (Prozac), and with tranquilizers to cause severe sedation. It has a double interaction with alcohol. People who drink while taking clonidine may have low blood pressure and also have much more sedation than would usually be caused by alcohol alone. Aldomet can interact with digitalis drugs to slow the heartbeat. It also interacts with some antidepressants, causing a rise in blood pressure.

Prazosin's effectiveness is lowered in people who take estrogen or anti-inflammatory medications such as ibuprofen. It strongly interacts with verapamil, causing low blood pressure and severe postural hypotension. Minoxidil can interact with anesthetic drugs to cause severely lowered blood pressure during surgery. If you are to have surgery, make sure the anesthesiologist knows you are taking this medication.

Antidysrhythmic Drugs

Many of the drugs previously discussed are used to treat certain dysrhythmias. Many types of dysrhythmias require treatment with specific antidysrhythmic medication, however.

Actions and Indications

All these drugs act by altering the electrical activity of cells in the conducting pathways of the heart. This change in electrical activity makes certain types of dysrhythmia less likely to occur. Differences between the various drugs that make certain ones better for certain types of dysrhythmia. Determining which drug is best for a specific rhythm disturbance is a very complex problem. In most cases, however, two or three drugs are likely to have a beneficial effect. Usually a trial-and-error period is needed to decide which drug is best for a particular patient.

Commonly Used Antidysrhythmic Drugs

Quinidine (Cardioquin, Duraquin, Quinaglute, Quinidex, Quinalin) is probably the most widely used of these medications. It can be used to treat abnormal rhythms of the atria, such as atrial fibrillation or flutter, and abnormal rhythms of the ventricles, such as premature ventricular beats.

Procainamide (Procan SR, Pronestyl) is used almost as frequently as quinidine. It is primarily prescribed for abnormal rhythms of the ventricles. Disopyramide (Norpace, Norpace CR) is used similarly to quinidine and procainamide and is sometimes effective when neither of those medications work. It has more depressant effects on the heart, however, so it is not as appropriate for persons in heart failure.

Several other drugs are used primarily to treat ventricular dysrhythmias that do not respond to the drugs mentioned above. Phenytoin (Dilantin) is an antiseizure medication that can effectively treat some ventricular dysrhythmias. Mexilitine (Mexitil) and tocainide (Tonocard) are closely related drugs that are also used for this purpose. Propafenone (Rhythmol) has effects similar to the other drugs in this class.

Flecainide (Tambocor) and encainide are two closely related drugs that were originally used like mexilitine, tocainide, and propafenone.

Later studies, however, reported that these two drugs may be associated with an increased mortality rate. For this reason they are now used only in persons with severe dysrhythmias that fail to respond to the other drugs in this class.

Amiodarone (Cordarone) can effectively treat many different forms of dysrhythmia that do not respond to other therapies. It has frequent and sometimes severe side effects, however, so its use is usually reserved for people with life-threatening problems that do not respond to other drugs.

Precautions and Side Effects

Quinidine can cause several side effects, though most are not severe. Many people taking quinidine experience intestinal cramps and diarrhea, and a few have nausea and vomiting. These symptoms usually go away within three weeks after starting the medication. Less common side effects include fever and rash, usually caused by an allergic reaction. If you experience these symptoms, you should call your doctor immediately. In some cases this allergic reaction can destroy the platelets (small structures in the blood that help stop bleeding). Occasionally, ringing in the ears, dizziness, and muscle or joint pain may occur.

Procainamide can cause rapid heartbeat or the symptoms of heart failure in a very few people. If you develop such symptoms you should be taken to a hospital immediately. A few people experience an allergic reaction to procainamide, including rash, chest or joint pain, and blisters. If you develop such symptoms, contact your doctor and stop taking the medication.

Disopyramide can worsen congestive heart failure symptoms in patients with weakened heart muscles. If this occurs, the drug must be discontinued and another substituted. The drug often causes dry mouth and difficulty urinating. If you experience these effects you should call your doctor. They can be treated easily and effectively. A few people also experience blurred vision or nausea.

Phenytoin may cause confusion, slurred speech, and difficulty balancing. These symptoms usually mean that the dose is too high. They will usually stop once the dose is lowered. A few people experience nausea or a measleslike rash. Phenytoin can interfere with the bone marrow's ability to produce blood cells, so your doctor will probably check your blood count a month or two after you start the medication.

Mexilitine and tocainide cause few side effects other than stomach upset. Some persons report they develop a slight tremor in their hands when taking these medicines, however. Tocainide, like phenytoin, may interfere with the bone marrow. Propafenone often causes mild dizziness, blurred vision, stomach upset, and changes in taste when first started. All these side effects usually resolve over time. A few patients develop asthma symptoms while taking propafenone. If this occurs, the medication should be discontinued.

Amiodarone often causes skin rashes and may cause a bluish or reddish discoloration of the skin. Sleep disturbance, headache, and muscle weakness are also common. Most people who take amiodarone for a long time will develop spots in their cornea (the clear part of the eye) that can interfere with vision. Nerve damage, resulting in weakness and numbness, can also occur and is sometimes permanent. Amiodarone can also interfere with the function of the thyroid gland and the liver. A rare but severe complication of amiodarone is the development of pulmonary alveolitis. This is a severe lung disease that causes scar tissue to develop throughout the lungs.

Interactions with Other Drugs

Quinidine is quite likely to interfere with the absorption of other medications. Usually this causes the patient to get less of the quinidine than usual and to absorb too much of the other medication. Procainamide can interact with certain antibiotics (called aminoglycosides) to cause severe muscle weakness. If you are taking procainamide, be certain to inform any doctor who might prescribe antibiotics for you. Disopyramide is likely to interact with antihypertensive medications, resulting in a much lower blood pressure. Usually the dose of antihypertensive medicine will have to be reduced.

Phenytoin also interacts with many different drugs. It increases the effects and side effects of antidepressants, tranquilizers, and digitalis preparations. Phenytoin reduces the effectiveness of cortisone, thyroid supplements, and oral diabetic medications. Cimetidine (Tagamet) can raise the levels of phenytoin, causing toxicity and increasing side effects. Cimetidine has a similar effect on mexilitine and tocainide. Tocainide can also interact with beta-blocking drugs, causing new dysrhythmias to develop. Beta blockers and tocainide should probably never be taken together.

Propafenone interacts with digitalis, beta blockers, and anticoagulants (blood-thinning medications), causing these medicines to increase their actions, which may result in toxic side effects. Flecainide can also increase the activity of digitalis and beta blockers, but not anticoagulants. Persons taking flecainide should not take antacids, since these can increase flecainide absorption and cause toxicity.

Medications to Lower Lipid and Cholesterol Levels

This is a broad category of medications. Unlike most of the other groups discussed, the medications used for this purpose have different actions and effects. For this reason, there are several subgroups of medications within this category. Some of these lower cholesterol generally, others lower LDL cholesterol, and others reduce triglycerides.

Actions and Indications

Most of the medications used to lower lipids and cholesterol work by methods that are not really understood, or at least not understood well. Two exceptions to this are bile acid sequestrants and enzyme inhibitors.

Bile acid sequestrants chemically bind bile in the intestines, removing the bile from the body. Since bile is very high in cholesterol, this eventually reduces blood cholesterol levels. Enzyme inhibitors block enzymes in the body that manufacture cholesterol and lipoproteins, reducing the amounts of cholesterol and triglycerides in the blood.

These medications are usually used when diet changes and exercise do not sufficiently reduce lipids and cholesterol in the blood to safe levels. In people who have severe elevations of cholesterol or lipids, they may be used immediately in addition to diet changes. They are also indicated in people who have hereditary conditions that cause elevated cholesterol or triglycerides.

Bile Acid Sequestrants

Bile acid sequestrants include cholestyramine (Questran, Cholybar) and colestipol (Colestid). These medications are prepared as powders to be mixed with beverages or food, or as chewable bars eaten with meals. Because these medications all cause bile acids to be passed through the entire intestine, rather than be reabsorbed, they can cause stomach upset. Most people experience symptoms including gas, abdominal cramps, and constipation when they begin taking these medications, but the symptoms usually stop after a few weeks.

The bile acid sequestrants are likely to bind other medications you take by mouth, preventing your body from absorbing them. For this reason, you should not take any medications for the period from one hour before to six hours after a dose of bile acid sequestrant. Even with proper precautions, bile acid sequestrants are likely to interfere with the absorption of other medications, and for that reason many doctors try not to use them.

When they are used, however, bile acid sequestrants usually result in a drop of serum cholesterol of 10 to 20 percent. They do not affect the levels of triglycerides, nor do they change the proportions of HDL and LDL cholesterol.

Enzyme-Blocking Agents

Several of these drugs interfere with an enzyme called HMG-CoA reductase. Blocking this enzyme allows the body to rid itself of cholesterol and also lowers the levels of LDL (bad) cholesterol and triglycerides (fats). The commonly used drugs of this type include lovastatin (Mevacor), pravastatin (Pravachol), and simvastatin (Zocor). All these are taken in pill form.

These medications are likely to cause mild muscle pain, weakness, and headache at first. These symptoms are usually mild and clear in a week or two in most cases, but occasionally they are severe. They may also cause blurred vision, headaches, stomach upset, and insomnia in a few cases. They may also interfere with liver function, so your doctor will probably order blood tests after you take this type of medication for a few weeks and repeat the tests every six weeks or so for the next year. The doctor may also send you for an annual eye examination, since a few people report eye trouble while taking these medications.

All these drugs can interfere with medications that prevent the blood from clotting, such as warfarin. If you are taking this medication, your doctor should test your blood clotting regularly to determine if there has been any change.

Niacin (Nia-Bid, Nicobid, Nicolar, Slo-Niacin, Nicotinex Elixir) inhibits different enzymes. The major effect of this drug is to lower triglycerides, but it also lowers LDL cholesterol and may raise HDL (good) cholesterol. Many of these drugs come in long-acting, time-release tablets. It is important to not crush or break the tablet, since this would release all the drug at once.

Most people report feeling warm and flushed for a short time after taking niacin, though most people don't find the feeling particularly unpleasant. A few people experience an unpleasant itch along with the flushed feeling. These sensations can be minimized by starting at a low dose of niacin and gradually increasing it. Alternatively, you can take one aspirin thirty minutes before taking the niacin to prevent this reaction.

Niacin causes few side effects, though some people experience mild headaches or stomach upset when they start the medication. In a very few cases, niacin interferes with liver functions, so your doctor may order blood tests a month or two after you've begun the medication.

Other Medications

Clofibrate (Atromid-S) is a medication used to lower triglycerides in the blood, although no one understands exactly how it works. To a lesser extent, it also lowers cholesterol levels. Clofibrate is often used for people who have genetically high triglyceride levels.

Many people have muscle pain and weakness when they first take clofibrate, but this usually clears up in a few weeks. People taking the drug must have periodic blood tests for liver function, since it can interfere with the liver. It has also been reported to cause gallstones and pancreatitis (inflammation of the pancreas) in a few people when taken for prolonged periods.

Gemfibrozil (Lopid) also lowers triglycerides by an unknown mechanism. Although it does not appear to lower total cholesterol, it raises the levels of HDL cholesterol in the blood. The side effects of gemfibrozil are similar to those of the enzyme-blocking drugs: muscle pain, blurred vision, insomnia, headaches, and stomach upset. It does not appear to cause any difficulty with white blood cells.

Two other cholesterol-reducing medications, probucol and dextrothyroxine, are rarely used in people with heart disease, because they can worsen cardiac problems. In a few cases, however, doctors may decide that lowering cholesterol is worth this risk.

Chapter 9

SURGERY AND ANGIOPLASTY

If this chapter had been written during the early 1960s, it would have been just a few pages long. At that time, open-heart surgery was rarely performed and usually was considered a last resort for people with terminal heart problems. The advent of the heart-lung bypass machine in the late 1950s made open-heart surgery feasible. The open-heart surgical procedures we take for granted today were developed throughout the 1960s. An explosion in the number of cardiac surgical procedures occurred during the 1970s and continued through the 1980s. Today, cardiac surgery is performed more frequently than appendectomy.

Advances in techniques and procedures made cardiac surgery the most rapidly expanding field of medicine throughout the 1970s. Operations were developed to treat conditions that had been considered incurable less than a decade before. Cardiac surgery probably reached its peak, at least in the number of procedures performed, during the early 1990s. In the rest of this decade, advancement has centered on performing procedures by cardiac catheterization, avoiding surgery in many cases. At this time, however, cardiac surgery is performed almost as frequently as it was a few years ago.

Although there is no question that these advances have improved the quality of treatment of heart disease patients in general, the large number of treatment options can result in confusion and controversy in the case of an individual patient. There are currently several different ways to treat coronary artery disease, for example. Coronary bypass surgery may be performed using a vein graft, an arterial graft, or both. Alternatively, angioplasty (dilating a diseased artery during a heart catheterization) may be performed by any of several methods, and a stent may or may not be left in place. New drugs developed to treat angina may allow either procedure to be delayed for months or years, or even avoided entirely.

The sheer number of treatment options has led to disagreements among doctors, especially between the specialties of cardiology and cardiac surgery, concerning what type of treatment is best in specific situations. Disagreements arise between doctors and insurance carriers about when and by what methods patients should be treated. It is not unusual for a patient to receive a second opinion that contradicts the first opinion, resulting in a third opinion that does not agree completely with either of the other two. Because of this situation, it is very important that you understand what the various surgical procedures are, what risks and benefits each has, and when they are indicated. If you want the best care possible, it is necessary that you become an informed consumer and make the decisions that are best for you.

Generally, when we talk about cardiac surgery we are speaking of "open-heart" procedures, where the heart itself is operated on and its structure altered. In the majority of cases, such surgery involves use of a heart-lung machine to take over the heart's pumping activity while the heart is operated on.

Many procedures that once required open-heart surgery can now be performed during a cardiac catheterization. Chapter 7 describes the catheterization procedure, since catheterization is usually performed for the diagnosis of heart disease. In this chapter, we will discuss what corrective procedures can be performed by catheterization and when they are indicated.

Before you have surgery, your doctor should explain what condition the procedure is going to treat, what the risks and benefits of the procedure are, and what the procedure and recovery will be like. This chapter provides an overview of what the different types of heart operations are used to treat, when they are indicated, and what results can be expected. The chapter also describes what patients experience before and immediately after the procedure. Chapter 10 will further describe the postsurgery recovery period.

Coronary Artery Bypass Graft Surgery

Coronary artery bypass graft surgery (often abbreviated CABG, and referred to as "cabbage" by doctors) is used to treat significant coronary artery disease. The principle of the procedure is simple. A healthy blood vessel is taken from some other part of the body and grafted from the aorta to the heart. The grafted vessel can then provide blood flow to the coronary arteries "downstream" from the area of blockage. CABG is the most common type of heart surgery performed today, with over 300,000 procedures performed each year in the United States.

Classically, a vein from the leg (the saphenous vein on the inside of the calf) is taken to use as the graft blood vessel. (There are several alternative veins in the leg, so removing the saphenous vein usually causes no problems.) One end of the vein is connected to the aorta near the heart, and the other end is connected to the diseased coronary artery. Since the atherosclerotic plaques usually occur in the first part of the coronary artery, the graft allows blood to flow normally through the rest of the artery, providing good circulation to the heart muscle.

In some cases, instead of using a vein to provide blood flow, an artery from the inside of the chest wall (the internal mammary artery) is used as the graft. The artery is dissected away from the chest and its end is sewn into the diseased coronary artery. (Since the chest wall receives blood from several other arteries, removing the internal mammary artery causes no problems.) It is technically more difficult to remove the internal mammary artery than it is to remove a vein, but there is some evidence that these grafts last longer than vein grafts. Only one internal mammary artery can be used, however, so when more than one graft is required (as is usually the case), vein grafts have to be used.

There are five major branches of the coronary arteries (Figure 9-1). Depending on the number of arteries that are diseased, as many as five separate grafts may be needed to restore normal circulation to the heart. In order for the surgeon to sew the grafts in place properly, it is necessary for the heart to stop beating. A heart-lung machine takes over the pumping function of the heart while the grafts are sewn into the aorta and coronary arteries.

Indications and Contraindications

The general indication for performing a coronary bypass is simple: Whenever one of the coronary arteries is obstructed to the point that it cannot deliver enough blood to the heart, it should be bypassed. The coronary arteries can dilate around an atherosclerotic plaque and still deliver a normal blood flow until the plaque has blocked off 50 percent of the artery's lumen (opening). At this degree of blockage people often experience angina during heavy exertion. Once the plaque has blocked 75 percent of the artery's lumen, the blood flow is not sufficient to supply the heart muscle during even minor exertion. People with this degree of blockage often experience angina even at rest.

As a general rule, when an artery is 75 percent occluded it should be treated either with bypass surgery or angioplasty (discussed later). Arteries that are less than 50 percent occluded should not be treated with surgery; the symptoms from this degree of blockage can usually be managed with medical therapy. Arteries that are between 50 and 75 percent occluded are usually treated if the patient's symptoms suggest the risk of a heart attack, if a stress test shows a lot of ischemia (lack of blood flow to the heart) during exercise, or if medical therapy does not relieve the symptoms.

The indications for bypass surgery also depend to some extent on which of the coronary arteries are involved in the disease. The left main coronary (Figure 9-1) provides the majority of blood flow to the entire heart, especially the left ventricle, in most people. Since obstruction of this artery almost always causes a massive heart attack resulting in death, surgeons are very likely to recommend bypass whenever the left main coronary artery has even 50 percent occlusion.

The left main coronary divides into the left anterior descending and the circumflex coronary arteries (Figure 9-1). Disease in both of these arteries is called "left main equivalent" disease and is also treated aggressively. Disease that is located more distally (further out in the circulation) is not as likely to cause a deadly heart attack, and doctors are more likely to recommend medical treatment.

Even when there is significant coronary disease, bypass surgery may not be possible. Bypass is only possible in the larger parts of the coronary arteries. If atherosclerotic disease involves the small distal parts of the arteries, bypass cannot be performed. Coronary bypass is less likely to work in people who have diabetes and in those with angina caused in part by hypertension. If a person has venous thromboembolism—that is, diseased veins that are clotting in their legs—taking the saphenous vein for a graft may worsen the circulation problems.

Although these principles concerning when bypass surgery is indicated seem fairly straightforward, they can be quite complicated to put into practice. The amount of obstruction in a vessel can only be estimated by angiography (see chapter 7), so different doctors may disagree

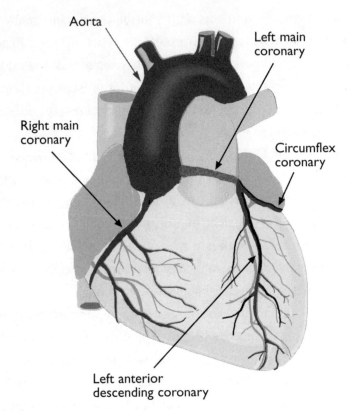

Figure 9-1: *The major branches of the coronary arteries.*

about how much blockage is present. The results of stress tests, nuclear medicine scans, and especially a patient's description of the symptoms may also be interpreted differently by different doctors. Even when the test results clearly indicate that some treatment is required, often a lot of discussion and debate occur about which treatment is most appropriate.

Unfortunately, many patients with coronary artery disease find themselves caught in this "bypass/don't bypass" debate. For some patients, the debate never reaches their ears but goes on behind the scenes. With the many changes that have occurred in the administration of health care in general, and the treatment for heart disease in specific, it is vitally important that you understand the forces influencing the decision of whether to operate on your heart.

Currently, coronary bypass surgery is performed over 300,000 times per year in the United States, at a total cost of well over ten billion dollars. In fact, more than half of all the CABGs performed in the world are done in the United States. In addition, about 400,000 Americans undergo angioplasty each year, at a cost of about five billion dollars. Similarly, only 200,000 angioplasties are performed in the rest of the world each year.

Needless to say, American insurance companies are trying very hard to reduce the number of these procedures. Some carriers, especially health maintenance organizations (groups that employ their own doctors to provide care), have strict criteria for when they will allow the procedure to be performed. It has been reported that given the same symptoms and disease, a patient participating in an HMO is only about half as likely to have bypass surgery recommended as one who is covered by either standard insurance or Medicare.

On the other hand, financial pressures can also affect doctors. One large review study published in the *Journal of the American Medical Association* found that almost 25 percent of bypass operations are not truly medically indicated. This does not mean that people with no coronary artery disease received bypass surgery, but rather that the patients had coronary disease that could have been managed safely with medication. This study was performed in the mid-1980s, however, and there is evidence that "unnecessary" bypass surgery is much less common today.

The important point of this discussion is that it is necessary to be an informed health-care consumer. You should know which coronary arteries are diseased and how significant the amount of blockage is. Ask the doctor what medical therapy has been tried, and if there are other alternatives. Any time bypass surgery is mentioned, ask for a second opinion regardless of whether your doctor or insurance company recommends one. A second opinion usually does not involve further tests; rather a second doctor reviews the tests that have been performed and either agrees or disagrees with the conclusions the original doctor reached. Almost every insurance plan will pay for a second opinion. In fact, many require it before any surgical procedure is performed.

What to Expect Before Surgery

The treatment you receive before open-heart surgery is generally the same whether the surgery involves coronary bypass or another type of procedure. Depending on how urgent your condition is, the procedure may be scheduled several weeks in advance or may be done the day after your condition is discovered. (Emergency bypass surgery, done during an actual heart attack, is discussed separately below.) Anyone who is about to have bypass surgery is anxious, and many people request a mild tranquilizer or sleeping pill to take for the few days before surgery. If you find yourself having such difficulties, tell your doctor so he or she can prescribe something appropriate for you.

During the period before surgery, your doctor may want you to avoid anti-inflammatory medications such as aspirin, ibuprofen (Motrin or Advil), or arthritis medicine since these can interfere with the blood's clotting ability. It isn't always necessary to stop these medications, but be sure your doctor knows if you're taking them during this time. Acetaminophen (Tylenol and most nonaspirin pain relievers) usually does not interfere with clotting, so it can be taken until the time of surgery without causing problems.

You should continue taking all other medications on schedule until you are admitted to the hospital, which will usually be the night before surgery. It is important that you report any changes in your symptoms to your doctor at this time, and also that you let the doctor know if you have any cold or flu symptoms or have been running any fever.

Because the heart-lung machine requires a significant amount of blood to work properly, almost everyone having bypass surgery will require blood transfusions. It is often possible for you to donate one or two units of your own blood to be used during surgery if you have several weeks' notice. If you are in good health, you can donate up to one unit of blood per week, and it can be stored for five weeks. Family members can also donate blood designated for your use if their blood type is compatible. Although people have contracted AIDS and hepatitis from blood transfusions in the past, modern screening methods make this risk very, very low. The risk of getting AIDS from a transfusion is now well less than one in a million.

Once you are admitted to the hospital, you will be visited and examined by your cardiologist, a member of the surgical team, an anesthesiologist, and a nurse. Each will do a brief examination, fill out routine history and physical forms, and answer any questions you have. The surgeon and anesthesiologist, in particular, should explain the procedure and advise you of the possible risks before you sign an "informed consent" for the surgery. A nurse or technician will also shave most of the hair from your body (to reduce the risk of infection) and will ask you to shower with antibacterial soap the night before surgery.

You will not be allowed to eat or drink anything for eight hours prior to surgery, although you will usually continue to take your medications as scheduled with a sip of water. Most surgeons will order a sedative if you need it, but generally it will only be given if you ask for it.

The morning of surgery, you will be asked to remove all clothes and jewelry and dress in a hospital gown. You will be taken to the preoperative holding area. (In a few hospitals you may be taken directly to the operating room.) The anesthesiologist will meet you there and start an intravenous line (IV) in your forearm. At that time, a sedative or pain medication can be given through the IV, if you need it.

The operating room may seem slightly intimidating. Usually at least half a dozen medical people will be present—nurses, orderlies, a technician who runs the heart-lung machine, other members of the surgical team—and all will be busy. The attention of the anesthesiologist and an assisting nurse will be focused entirely on you, however. If you are nervous or uncomfortable, let them know.

Once you have been moved onto the operating table, the anesthesiologist will connect you to an EKG machine, blood pressure cuff, and one or two other monitors. You will also be asked to breathe oxygen through a face mask. The anesthesiologist will start a second IV in your other arm and will usually insert an arterial line (a small catheter inserted in the artery near your wrist) before you receive anesthesia. You will be given a local anesthetic before insertion of the catheters, so they shouldn't hurt at all. Once all the monitors have been tested and shown to function, the anesthesiologist will let you know you are going to sleep. The anesthesia is given through your IV, so there will be no smelly gases to breathe.

The Surgical Procedure

After the anesthesia has taken effect, the anesthesiologist will usually insert a central venous catheter or pulmonary artery catheter into the large vein below your collarbone or at the base of your neck (see chapter 7). A breathing tube will be inserted through your mouth into your windpipe to allow a ventilator to breathe for you. This tube will be left in place for several hours or even a day or more after surgery. It is not uncomfortable, but it will prevent you from talking when you first wake up.

The surgeon will make an incision down the center of your chest through the breastbone to expose the heart. Another incision will be made on the inside of one leg to remove the saphenous vein to use for the grafts. In some cases, a third incision is made along one side of the groin to connect the heart-lung machine. Usually the machine is connected directly to the large blood vessels in the chest, however.

Once the vein has been removed and the heart-lung machine connected, the surgeon will begin sewing in the bypass grafts. Depending on the number of grafts and how much atherosclerosis exists in the coronary arteries, this can take from one to three hours. Once the grafts are in place, your heart will be allowed to start pumping again, assisted by the heart-lung machine. After the surgeon is comfortable that all the grafts are functioning and your heart is working well, the heart-lung machine is turned off and disconnected. The breastbone is sewn back together with surgical wires, and all the incisions are closed using sutures and staples.

Unlike other surgical procedures, you will not wake up in the operating room. While you are still under anesthesia, the surgical team will transport you to the intensive care unit and connect you to all the monitors and ventilators there. The anesthesia is allowed to wear off slowly, and you will usually not wake up for an hour or more after you get to the ICU.

When you first wake up, it is important to remember that you are connected to a lot of equipment. An endotracheal tube—a tube that goes through your mouth and into your windpipe—will allow a mechanical ventilator to breathe for you. You can still take breaths on your own, but the ventilator makes sure you get enough oxygen. Most of the time the endotracheal tube will be removed within three to twelve hours.

There will also be several IVs and an arterial line, a central venous catheter, and a catheter to empty your bladder. Some plastic tubes will be inserted into your chest cavity to drain any fluid or blood that collects there after the surgery. The catheters and tubes will be removed over the next two or three days.

While all this can be a bit overwhelming, the tubes are not painful. They will make it difficult for you to move around much without assistance, however. At any rate, you will be heavily sedated for the first twelve to twenty-four hours after surgery, so you may not even remember this phase of your postoperative care.

For the Family During Surgery

After open-heart surgery the patient is taken to the intensive care unit rather than back to an ordinary hospital room. After your family member has been taken to the operating room, a member of the nursing staff will help you gather any personal possessions from the room and take you to the ICU waiting room. The operating room staff will contact you there later. The waiting room usually has a volunteer host or hostess who will be happy to take messages for you or forward calls to you if you want to go to the cafeteria or take a walk.

Most families are very concerned with how long the surgical procedure will take. It is important to remember that a lot of activity has to take place before the surgery even begins. Often family members begin wondering "are they done yet?" before the surgery has even started. Most operating rooms send for their patients at least forty-five minutes before they are ready to begin surgery. As a general rule, it takes another thirty minutes to perform all the preliminaries—monitoring, starting IVs, inducing anesthesia—before the surgery starts. If everything moves very rapidly, the surgery may begin an hour after the patient has left for the operating room, but it is often closer to two hours.

Once the surgery begins, a surgical nurse will usually call the waiting room to let you know they've started. During this first call, the nurse should tell you how often the OR will call back. Each hospital has its own protocol for keeping family members informed, but most will either call you every hour or will call you when the bypass grafts have been connected and the heart-lung machine turned off. If the nurse doesn't say when they will call back, be sure to ask. You can also ask the hostess to check with the operating room if you don't hear from the nurse as scheduled.

The intensive care unit nurses will also call the waiting room when your family member has arrived in the ICU. Usually they will need an hour or so to get all the monitors connected, give medications, and perform any lab tests the surgeon has ordered. During this time, the surgeon will probably come by the ICU waiting room to talk with you and let you know how the surgery went and what to expect for the next twelve hours or so. By the time the surgeon has left, the ICU nurses will usually let you in to visit for a few minutes, although it is unlikely that your family member will be awake yet.

Be prepared to be a little overwhelmed during your first ICU visit. Your family member will be surrounded by a lot of beeping or flashing monitoring equipment. Several tubes and intravenous lines will be connected to various devices around the bed. Most importantly, the patient will be connected to a ventilator and will not be able to talk. If the patient has had time to completely wake up, he or she will be able to write notes and can hear you perfectly well. This is all routine, and the majority of the monitors and tubes, as well as the ventilator, will usually be removed within twenty-four hours.

After this first visit, you can return during the regular ICU visiting hours, which are posted in the waiting room. Unless there is an overwhelming reason, you should not ask to visit outside of the usual visiting hours. The ICU is a very busy place, and it is difficult for the nurses to "work around" a visitor.

The Expected Outcomes and Possible Complications of CABG

The purpose of bypass surgery is to restore normal blood flow to the heart, reducing or eliminating the symptoms of coronary artery disease. About 90 percent of patients who undergo CABG report a dramatic improvement in their symptoms, with angina attacks eliminated altogether or markedly reduced in frequency and severity. About 80 percent of patients report that their activity level increases once they have recovered from surgery, and about half report improvement in other symptoms such as shortness of breath or swelling.

The ability of CABG to actually prolong life has been demonstrated only in one group of patients, however. People who have left main coronary artery disease or left main equivalent disease will definitely live longer if they undergo CABG. Other studies show that people with more than 75 percent blockage in at least two separate coronary arteries, who also have impaired pumping function of their heart, will also have a longer life expectancy if they have CABG, but not all studies agree. For persons with coronary artery disease involving other vessels, CABG can effectively improve the symptoms but has not been shown to prolong life any more than careful medical management.

The underlying disease of atherosclerosis is not changed by a bypass procedure. About half of all persons who have a CABG will have new coronary artery disease within ten years after the procedure. The incidence is much higher in those who don't make lifestyle changes to lower their risk factors. New atherosclerotic plaques can form in the coronary arteries or in the vein grafts used to bypass existing plaques.

Of course, the benefit of CABG is not without risk. The perioperative (during and after surgery) mortality of CABG is about 3 to 4 percent. Persons who have well-controlled angina and undergo the procedure electively have a lower mortality rate. Those who have emergency CABG, are undergoing the procedure for a second time, or have other medical diseases (such as diabetes, hypertension, pulmonary disease) have a higher mortality rate.

About 2 percent of persons who undergo CABG will develop some type of complication. Any operation involving the blood vessels can result in some postoperative bleeding, which may require a second operation. Usually such operations are minor procedures compared to the CABG itself. Another 5 percent of people will actually suffer a heart attack during or immediately after the procedure. These are usually small heart attacks that were probably caused by a bit of plaque being chipped off during surgery and flowing downstream to block a small branch of a coronary artery. In most cases, such attacks do not interfere with post-operative recovery.

About 10 to 20 percent of patients undergoing CABG report some neurologic (brain and nerve) problems after surgery. The most commonly reported symptoms are irritability, insomnia, restlessness, and forgetfulness. It is believed, although not known for certain, that small amounts of air introduced into the bloodstream by the heart-lung machine cause these effects on brain function after surgery. In the majority of cases the symptoms go away within a month or two. In recent years, new drugs have been administered just before starting the heart-lung machine, in an effort to eliminate these effects. It is not yet known for certain whether they are of benefit.

Angioplasty

Angioplasty is another way to restore blood flow through a coronary artery that is blocked by plaque. The procedure is performed by cardiac catheterization, in which a catheter is placed in an artery and threaded through the aorta and into the coronary artery using X-ray guidance. The complete name for the procedure is percutaneous (throughout the skin) transluminal (within the blood vessel) coronary angioplasty (repair of the blood vessel), usually abbreviated PTCA.

PTCA was developed in the 1980s. It was originally thought that PTCA would almost completely replace CABG surgery, but that has not yet occurred. PTCA is now performed more frequently than CABG, however, and is often used as an alternative. There continues to be a lot of debate concerning when PCTA is indicated and how effective it is.

The Angioplasty Procedure

The preparation for PTCA is similar to that for CABG surgery, although the procedure is more likely to be performed on an outpatient basis. As with any major procedure, you should not eat or drink for eight hours before the procedure, except to take your medicine with a sip of water. Once you are admitted to the hospital, the cardiologist will discuss the procedure and obtain your informed consent in writing.

The angioplasty is performed in the coronary angiography suite rather than the operating room. You will remain awake during the procedure but will be given a sedative and some strong pain medicine before it begins. The major parts of the procedure are identical to those for cardiac catheterization (see chapter 7). In fact, your cardiologist may get permission to do angioplasty during your first catheterization, just in case there is a need to perform it. The catheterization itself is not painful, although you may feel some pressure in the area of the groin where the catheters are inserted.

Once the angioplasty catheter has been placed near the area of blockage, the cardiologist will tell you that the angioplasty is about to begin. The most commonly performed type is balloon angioplasty, which uses a catheter that has a small, inflatable balloon tip. Once the catheter is placed in the area of blockage the balloon is inflated, stretching the artery and flattening the plaque.

The balloon is usually inflated for thirty to sixty seconds, then deflated. During the time the catheter is inflated the artery is entirely obstructed, so you may experience some angina. Be sure to tell the cardiologist if this occurs (the doctor will probably ask you anyway). A series of two or three inflations is performed, followed by an X ray to see how much the blockage has been improved.

Other methods are sometimes used to perform PTCA besides the balloon catheter method. Some catheters are designed to actually cut out the plaque (known as an atherectomy), while others use laser beams to burn the plaque away. Neither method has been shown to be more effective than balloon angioplasty in large clinical trials, but there is some hope that their success rates may eventually be superior to the balloon method. From a patient's viewpoint, however, the procedure is the same whatever method is used.

In some cases, the cardiologist may choose to leave a stent, a spring-shaped piece of surgical metal that is expected to hold the artery open and prevent blockage from recurring. Although they increase the odds of a vessel remaining open, stents are associated with a slightly higher complication rate. For this reason they are often reserved for especially large plaques or high-risk areas of the arteries.

The entire angioplasty procedure will take from one to three hours, depending on the number of coronary vessels that must be treated. After the procedure you may be monitored in the angiography suite or a nearby recovery room for an hour or two. Following this you are transferred to a coronary monitored bed—that is, one that has twenty-four-hour EKG monitoring. This will usually not be in an ICU, but rather on a "coronary care" floor of the hospital. Most people will remain hospitalized overnight. You can eat or drink as soon as you return to the room.

The sheath that was placed in the artery in your groin will be left in place for anywhere from two to twenty-four hours following the procedure. Once it has been removed, a pressure dressing will be placed on the area for about twenty-four hours. During the time the sheath is in place, and for six hours after it is removed, you should not bend your leg or try to stand up because this could cause bleeding at the puncture site. The nurses will tell you when you can sit in a chair or walk.

Family members will often be allowed to stay in your hospital room while you have angioplasty, although they may be moved to a waiting room if you are going to a different floor after the procedure. The staff from the angioplasty suite will call after the angioplasty has been completed, and the cardiologist will usually come by the room to talk to family members before you have arrived back from the recovery area.

Most people return home the day after their PTCA. While you should definitely take it easy for two or three days after the procedure, most people are able to return to work within ten days. Usually you will have a follow-up stress test or arteriogram three to six months after angioplasty.

The Expected Outcomes and Possible Complications of PTCA

About 90 percent of patients who undergo PTCA will have a reduction in the number and severity of angina attacks. Most of these patients will also report an improvement in their activity level and are able to reduce the amount of medication they take for angina. No studies have shown an overall increase in life expectancy following angioplasty, however. This may be explained in part because most persons with "left main" disease undergo CABG rather than angioplasty.

The major difference in outcome between angioplasty and CABG is in how long the improvement lasts. Slightly less than 70 percent of initially successful PTCA patients are still angina free 6 months after the procedure, compared to more than 85 percent of CABG patients. In a significant number of patients treated by PTCA, the plaque returns to its original size within the first year after the procedure, requiring a repeat PTCA or a CABG.

On the other hand, the costs and risks involved with PTCA are clearly lower than those involved with CABG. A PTCA procedure costs less than one-third what a CABG does, and the recovery time is measured in days rather than weeks or months. The mortality rate for PTCA is less than

1 percent, and the chance of having a heart attack during the procedure is less than 4 percent. The mortality and heart attack rates are slightly higher for CABG procedures.

About 1 percent of persons who undergo PTCA will suffer a major complication such as rupture of the coronary artery or a sudden heart attack. In these cases it may be necessary to perform emergency cardiac surgery, usually including a CABG. In some hospitals, the cardiac surgeon who is available to "back up" the angioplasty procedure may meet with you before the angioplasty. This is routine and does not mean that doctors expect difficulty in your case.

Another 2 percent of people who undergo PTCA have a less serious or delayed complication. Most commonly this involves damage to the artery in the groin through which the catheterization was performed. Almost all such complications can be repaired, although surgery is usually required.

The Angioplasty-Versus-CABG Debate

When angioplasty first became widely used, controversy arose between cardiologists (who perform cardiac tests and angioplasty) and cardiac surgeons (who perform CABG) about the effectiveness of the procedure. The medical literature was filled with reports from both groups, some strongly advocating angioplasty for almost everyone with coronary artery disease, others saying the treatment was dangerous and ineffective.

Looking back on the initial reports, most doctors now agree that cardiologists were probably overaggressive in using angioplasty instead of surgery. Likewise, the procedure was more effective and had lower risks than cardiac surgeons initially claimed. During the 1990s, several large, long-term studies have been consolidated and are beginning to provide a much clearer picture of when a person should have angioplasty and when CABG is appropriate.

In summary, most of these studies agree that angioplasty has a lower risk of death, heart attack, and other complications than CABG does. Angioplasty can also be performed fairly safely in people who are too ill to undergo CABG. Patients who have angioplasty are more likely to have recurrence of their plaque than people who undergo CABG, and the recurrence often happens within a year or two, compared to four to six years later for those having CABG.

In general, most cardiologists recommend angioplasty whenever there is disease involving only one or two branches of the coronary artery, especially if the plaques are located close to the aorta. Some recommend angioplasty even when three or more branches are diseased. Although some cardiologists will try angioplasty on persons with left main coronary artery disease, only CABG has been shown to improve long-term survival in patients who have plaques in this location.

If angioplasty initially relieves symptoms of angina, but they recur in a few months or a year, the decision is less clear. Many cardiologists will then repeat angioplasty, often leaving a stent in place. Others feel that surgery should probably be performed in this situation. Certainly if two angioplasties have each given only short-term relief, a CABG is indicated.

It is always important to remember exactly what is expected from any type of invasive procedure, especially when it is performed to treat heart disease. Both angioplasty and CABG have been shown to decrease the symptoms of angina and improve the quality of life in people with coronary artery disease. Neither has been statistically shown to increase life expectancy, except for the treatment of left main coronary artery disease by CABG. However, most physicians believe that the statistics don't accurately separate out those people who make major lifestyle changes after surgery from those who don't. It seems logical to believe that if people truly reduce their coronary risk factors following surgery, many could avoid recurrence of their heart disease.

Surgery for Valvular Heart Disease

Most patients with valvular heart disease are treated medically and observed for worsening of their condition for several years before any further treatment is needed. For some conditions, techniques performed during cardiac catheterization called balloon valvuloplasty (literally "reshaping the valve") can be effective and allow patients to avoid open-heart surgery. For many other types of valvular disease, open-heart surgery will eventually be required.

Balloon valvuloplasty can be used for many people with pulmonary or mitral valve stenosis. In a few cases it is used for people who have aortic stenosis, but as a rule it is not as successful for treating this condition.

Undergoing balloon valvuloplasty is almost identical to undergoing an angioplasty (see above). Instead of a small balloon being used to dilate a coronary artery, however, a large balloon is used to stretch the stenotic valve, enlarging its opening. In almost all cases, significant improvement occurs following the procedure. If the diseased valve continues to worsen, however, surgery may be required some years later.

Most people will stay in the hospital only for a day or two after balloon valvuloplasty. Like any invasive procedure, it presents potential complications, but the incidence is quite low. There is a 1 to 2 percent possibility of damage to the valve during the procedure, which may require surgical replacement of the valve.

All the actual surgical procedures for valve disease are open-heart procedures. The preparations before surgery and the postoperative care are almost identical to those described above for coronary artery bypass surgery. The procedures themselves usually take about four to five hours to perform; it may take longer if more than one valve must be replaced.

The type of surgery performed depends on the type of valvular disease, how severe the disease is, and the age of the patient. When the valvular disease is not too severe, a surgical valvuloplasty may be attempted. Unlike balloon valvuloplasty, surgical valvuloplasty can mean enlarging the opening of a stenotic valve or using sutures to narrow and strengthen the opening of a regurgitating valve. Valvuloplasty is not performed for diseased aortic valves, because this valve is subjected to very high pressures that would break down the surgical repairs.

When a valve is severely diseased or has a lot of calcium deposited in the leaflets, it must be replaced with either a biological valve or a mechanical valve. Biological valves are animal or human heart valves that have been sterilized and treated to prevent rejection. Mechanical valves are made of titanium and plastic.

Biological valves have one advantage over mechanical valves—they do not cause blood clots, so the patient does not have to take anticoagulant medications after valve replacement. Biological valves are not as durable as artificial valves, however. About 40 percent of biological valves will require replacement ten years or so after they are implanted. Generally, biological valves are used for valve replacement in older people and for those who cannot take anticoagulant (blood-thinning) medications.

Mechanical valves are extremely durable and hardly ever need to be replaced. All mechanical valves cause a reaction in the blood, causing the blood to try to form clots around the valve. For this reason, persons having mechanical valves will have to take anticoagulant medication for the rest of their lives. These valves also make a clicking sound when they open and close, which may take a little while to get used to.

Having either type of replacement valve puts a person at high risk of developing endocarditis (inflammation of the heart's lining and valves). Because of this, people who have artificial valves will need to take antibiotics whenever they are exposed to a bacterial infection. The risk of developing endocarditis is no different than that for any person with a diseased heart valve, however.

Less Common Surgical Procedures

Heart Transplantation

Heart transplantation has become a fairly common procedure, with over 2,000 transplants performed in the United States each year. Because the number of donor hearts is very limited (30 percent of people awaiting heart transplants will die before a donor is available), the use of heart transplantation is strictly limited to those people who are most likely to benefit. The usual criteria for being considered a candidate for heart transplantation are: (1) irreversible heart disease; (2) a life expectancy of two years or less; and (3) age below sixty-five.

Persons who meet these criteria are then carefully screened to determine if they are a candidate. Persons who have other diseased organs that would significantly shorten life (kidney disease, for example), or have other life-shortening factors (such as significant obesity or continued smoking), will not be considered candidates. Likewise, those who have a disease that could be worsened by the immune-system-suppressing drugs that must be taken after a transplant cannot be considered candidates.

If a person meets all the criteria and has no contraindications, the transplant surgeon can declare the patient a candidate for heart transplant and have the person's name put on a waiting list for a donor heart. Once a person is on the waiting list, he or she must always be within two or three hours' travel time from the hospital where the transplant will take place. The person will be given a beeper so the hospital can reach the patient at any time.

Legally, transplants must be performed on a first come, first served basis. Exceptions can be made, however, if the transplant candidate becomes so ill that he or she must be hospitalized in an ICU and requires life-support methods. Those who receive a donor heart have an 85 to 90 percent chance of surviving the first year after the procedure. Survival rates are about 95 percent for each succeeding year.

The procedures immediately before a heart transplant are very similar to those for other open-heart surgery, although even more care is taken to make sure there is no exposure to any possible source of infection. The immediate postoperative recovery is also very similar, although patients will usually remain in protective isolation, since they are very vulnerable to infection at first. Family members and other visitors will be required to wear hospital gowns and masks whenever they are around the transplant recipient.

In addition to the type of treatment that follows any heart surgery, the transplant recipient will have to take medications to suppress the immune system so that it doesn't reject the donor heart. These medications are very individualized, meaning the dose has to be constantly monitored and adjusted during the first weeks after the transplant. Even after they go home from the hospital (usually about three weeks after the surgery), transplant recipients may have to wear a surgical mask in public places to avoid exposure to infection.

The drugs will also cause some weight gain and may cause mild diabetes, kidney problems, or high blood pressure. They also slightly increase the risk of developing certain types of cancer. Over time, however, the dose of medication can be decreased in many patients, and the severity of the side effects lessens.

Even with medication, there is always a risk that the immune system will begin attacking the donor heart tissue, a process known as rejection. In order to detect rejection, a heart transplant recipient will undergo several biopsies—removal of a tiny piece of the donor heart to be examined under a microscope. The biopsy is performed by inserting a catheter in the large vein under the collarbone and threading it into the heart, where a small bit of tissue is removed under X-ray guidance. Usually a biopsy is done every week for the first six weeks, then once a month for the next six months.

Pericardial Window

In a few people, the saclike membrane enclosing the heart, the pericardium, becomes filled with fluid. This may be caused by viral infection or by another disease involving the heart. In any case, the fluid surrounding the heart may accumulate to the point that it prevents the heart from functioning properly. In this situation, it becomes necessary to surgically open the pericardium and drain the fluid from it using a procedure called a pericardial window.

The procedure is surgically quite simple. However, it is necessary for the person having the procedure to remain awake for as long as possible, since general anesthesia interferes with the heart's ability to pump against the surrounding pressure. For this reason, a patient having a pericardial window performed will generally remain awake while the surgeon scrubs the area and applies all the surgical drapes. Once the surgeon is ready to operate, the anesthesiologist will administer the anesthetic and the procedure begins.

Following the procedure, the patient will have to stay in the recovery room for an hour or two. In most cases, the patient can return to the regular hospital floor without having to stay in the ICU. Almost everyone who has a pericardial window is dramatically improved after the surgery.

Emergency Procedures

Thrombolytic Therapy

The final event causing most heart attacks is the formation of a blood clot over a plaque in a coronary artery. The clot blocks whatever opening remains in the artery, and heart muscle downstream from the clot no longer receives any blood. The heart muscle's cells don't actually begin to die for thirty minutes to two hours after the blood flow is stopped, however, and if blood flow can be restored during this time, the heart muscle can recover fully without permanent damage.

Thrombolytic (clot-dissolving) drugs dissolve blood clots. If they are given to a heart attack victim soon enough, they can often reverse the attack. The thrombolytic drugs streptokinase and urokinase are obtained from natural sources and have been available for many years. The artificially produced thrombolytic drug tissue plasminogen activator (TPA) has been available since the early 1990s. When this drug was introduced, several studies claimed it was superior to the other drugs in its ability to dissolve the clots causing heart attack and stroke. Since that time, however, many studies have demonstrated that all these drugs are equally effective.

No matter which drug is used, the procedure of administering it is the same. The drugs are administered into an IV catheter as soon as the heart attack is diagnosed in the emergency room. The drug is given slowly over an hour or so, while the patient's EKG and other signs are monitored carefully. Eighty percent of heart attack victims who receive the drugs within two hours after their symptoms start will have reperfusion (restored blood flow) of the area involved in the heart attack. This does not mean that no permanent damage occurs, but it minimizes the amount of heart tissue that is damaged, reducing the size and severity of the attack.

If more than two hours have passed, the drugs give much less benefit. After four hours they have no beneficial effect and should not be used. Since the drugs will also dissolve blood clots in other parts of the body, they cannot be used in people who have had recent injuries or surgery, or those who have active stomach ulcers.

Emergency CABG

Emergency coronary bypass surgery is sometimes required for people who suffer massive heart attacks that don't respond to medical treatment. It may also be needed for a person who has a heart attack while undergoing angioplasty. The procedure, of course, is the same whether it takes place electively or as a sudden emergency. Because the condition of a person having emergency bypass surgery is usually much more serious, emergency bypass surgery carries a much higher risk than elective surgery.

Emergency CABG surgery can be expected to take longer than a similar procedure done electively. Because of the damage that occurred before surgery, the patient's heart often does not pump well after emergency CABG. In such a situation, it is not unusual for surgeons to insert an aortic balloon pump to help the patient's heart pump blood effectively.

The aortic balloon pump is a large balloon catheter that is inserted through the patient's groin into the aorta. The balloon is connected to a large external box that rapidly inflates and deflates the balloon in between the patient's own heartbeats. The inflating balloon serves as an accessory pump, helping the heart to move blood through the body and reducing the heart's workload. Balloon pumps can only be left in place for a few days, however. By that time the heart must be able to function on its own.

Although emergency CABG surgery has a high mortality rate (about 8 to 10 percent), it is the only hope for some people. Persons who survive the first few days after surgery have results similar to those who underwent an elective CABG.

Summary

Open-heart surgery provides hope of a normal life for many people who otherwise would have terminal heart disease. Following successful surgery, many people can perform their daily activities with almost no symptoms of heart disease. Open-heart surgery does carry significant risks and is never undertaken lightly, however.

It is important to realize that no cardiac surgical procedure is a "cure" for heart disease. The disease is still present, even though its severity and symptoms are often dramatically reduced after surgery. Unfortunately, too many people believe that since they've had such improvement, they are free of heart disease. They return to their previous high-risk lifestyle. Numerous studies have shown that doing so will quickly reverse the improvement gained by surgery. Those people who use surgery as a chance to make lifestyle changes to improve their heart's health are much more likely to keep the surgery's benefits for many years.

Chapter 10

THE POSTOPERATIVE
RECOVERY PERIOD

Recovery After Catheterization and Angioplasty

Following cardiac catheterization or angioplasty, you will be monitored in a post-catheterization care unit. In this area you will have very close nursing care, with each nurse assigned to no more than two patients. An EKG will monitor the electrical activity of your heart, and an automated blood pressure cuff will check your blood pressure every few minutes.

During the time you are in this unit, a complete 12-lead EKG will usually be run in addition to the standard monitoring EKG. This will be compared to your EKG from before the procedure to make sure you haven't suffered any damage to the heart muscle or conducting system. Some blood will be drawn to check your cardiac enzymes (see chapter 2) for the same reason.

During your stay the nurse will examine the artery in your groin every fifteen minutes or so to make sure there is no bleeding from the puncture site. The nurse will also perform neurovascular checks, making sure the pulses and sensation to the lower leg remain normal. You will probably be allowed to drink a little water while you are in the post-catheterization unit, but you will not be able to eat yet.

If you had a cardiac catheterization without angioplasty, you may remain in this unit for four hours or so and then be discharged home. The doctor will come and discuss the results of the angiography (X rays of the coronary arteries) with you before you leave and schedule a follow-up visit in a week or two. If only moderate narrowing of the coronary arteries was found, the doctor may prescribe some new medications before you go home.

If significant coronary disease was found, or if you had an angioplasty or other procedure performed, you will be transferred to a monitored bed after a one- or two-hour stay in the post-catheterization unit. Monitored beds have twenty-four-hour EKG monitoring by telemetry so that a monitor at the nurses' station always shows your EKG tracing. Depending on the facilities and space available at the hospital, this may be in the coronary care unit, or in a step-down unit (a unit with care that is "one step" below that of an ICU). Usually you will remain in the telemetry unit for about twenty-four hours.

Depending on the actual procedure you had and the severity of your disease, you may spend a few days in a standard hospital room after your stay in the telemetry unit, or you may be discharged home. After you get home, you should not walk long distances for a few days, in order to give the artery in your leg time to heal. If you notice any numbness or pain in the foot on the side your catheterization was performed on, you should call your doctor immediately.

Most people can return to work or resume normal activities within a week following a catheterization or angioplasty. Some bruising and soreness around the catheter site is normal, but it should clear up within a week to ten days.

Recovery After Open-Heart Surgery

Recovery following open-heart surgery is, of course, more prolonged than that following catheterization or angioplasty. Most people, however, resume most of their everyday activities within two months following open-heart surgery. A complete recovery may take three to four months.

The Immediate Recovery Period—The ICU

Following open-heart surgery, you will wake up in the intensive care unit. You will be immediately aware of the endotracheal tube, which passes through your mouth into your windpipe, and the mechanical ventilator. The sensation of a machine breathing for you takes a little while to get used to, and you will find it uncomfortable at first. It is important that you not fight the ventilator. Trying to resist the breaths it delivers will increase your discomfort. It is all right to take additional breaths between the ventilator breaths, however. The machine will deliver as much air as you want.

Because of the endotracheal tube, you will be unable to talk. The nurses will explain everything carefully to you and ask you to nod or squeeze their hand to show that you understand. They will also give you a pad and pencil to write down any questions or requests when you are awake enough to communicate. For most people, the ventilator will be disconnected after a few hours in the ICU, and you will be allowed to breathe on your own. If there are no problems, the endotracheal tube will be removed an hour or two later. You will need to wear an oxygen mask for a day or so after the endotracheal tube is removed.

You will also have an IV in one arm and an arterial line in the artery at your wrist, as well as a central venous catheter inserted under your collarbone or at the base of your neck. None of these catheters are painful, but it is important that you move slowly so that you don't pull them out. A urinary catheter will be in place to empty your bladder. This catheter may make it feel like you have to urinate, even though it is actually emptying your bladder. There will also be some plastic tubes that drain any fluid or blood that collects in your chest.

While all this is a bit overwhelming, the tubes are not painful. They will make it difficult for you to move around without assistance. You will be heavily sedated for the first twelve to twenty-four hours after surgery, however, so you probably won't need to move much. You may not even remember this phase of your postoperative care. Most of the tubes and catheters will be removed over the first two to three days after surgery.

Within a few hours after you've awakened, the nurses will probably try to get you to sit up in bed, or perhaps in a chair beside the bed. This may seem like cruel and unusual punishment to someone who has just had major surgery, but actually it's very important. Sitting up, even for only fifteen or twenty minutes, can help prevent pneumonia from beginning in your lungs and blood clots from forming in your legs. The nursing team is very experienced at helping people sit up after surgery. Let them take care of the various lines and tubes.

Because the surgery required the sternum (breastbone) to be split lengthwise, most people find it painful to use their arms for moving themselves around in bed. Usually it is not painful to push backward with your elbows, but you may find it difficult to push forward or downward with your arms and hands.

More importantly, you will probably find it painful to cough or take deep breaths after the breathing tube has been removed. It is extremely important that you do cough and breathe deeply after heart surgery, however. Failure to do so will often result in pneumonia and will require the endotracheal tube to be replaced and the ventilator reconnected.

The nurses will use a spirometer—a device that measures how deeply you breathe—every few hours to make sure you are breathing deeply enough. They will also show you how to use a pillow to press down on your sternum when you cough, preventing most of the pain. If you still find coughing extremely painful, however, make sure you ask for more pain medicine. It is vitally important that you breathe deeply and cough after this type of surgery.

Your heartbeat will be continuously monitored during your stay in the ICU. During surgery, the doctors usually put temporary pacemaker wires near your heart. If there is any need, a temporary pacemaker can be connected to these in a few seconds and take over pacemaker activity for your heart. This is not unusual during the first day after open-heart surgery, and a need for a temporary pacemaker does not mean a permanent pacemaker will be needed later.

All your nutrition will be received through intravenous lines for the first day or so after surgery. Once the doctors have determined that your bowels have returned to proper function, they will put you on a liquid diet. If you have no problems with that, you can start eating regular food.

By the second or third day after surgery, most of the tubes and lines will have been removed. Usually patients are able to sit up by themselves and walk with some assistance by this time. As you begin walking, you will probably be bothered more by the incision in your leg where the vein was removed than by the chest incision. Your leg will be kept wrapped in elastic bandages to ease this pain and to prevent swelling. Walking is very important, even if it is painful at first, because the muscles in the leg help pump blood through the veins whenever you walk. This can prevent the formation of blood clots in the remaining veins of your leg, one of the more frequent complications after CABG.

During your ICU stay, family members will be able to visit three or four times a day for fifteen to thirty minutes each time. Usually only two family members at a time will be allowed in, but some hospitals allow three. As your condition improves, you may be allowed to have a bed-side telephone, but this depends on the policies of the hospital.

Doctors often joke that the first sign of recovery after heart surgery is that the patients complain about being in the ICU. The ICU is a very busy and fairly noisy place. You may find it difficult to rest, especially after the first twenty-four hours when the anesthetic has completely worn off. Don't hesitate to ask for a sedative or pain medication if you need them. These are almost always ordered "as needed" by the surgeon, so they won't be given unless you ask for them.

Once you are able to walk a little and have had most of the tubes and lines removed, you will be transferred to a regular hospital bed—usually about the third day after surgery. If you have had no dysrhythmias during your ICU stay, you may be able to go directly to a regular postoperative floor. In most cases, however, the surgeon will have you transferred to a monitored bed in a "step-down" unit. In either case, family members can now visit during regular visiting hours, and usually your spouse can stay overnight in the room if you desire.

The Intermediate Recovery Period—Step-Down or Monitored Care

The step-down care unit or monitored care unit looks much more like an ordinary hospital room than the ICU did. It is different from a regular hospital floor in that the nurses are specially trained, and there are more nurses available. Each patient also is attached to an EKG monitor at all times. The EKG tracing is visible in the room, and a continuous display is also shown on a monitor at the nurses' station. One nurse is always watching the monitors to make sure no patient is having rhythm problems. Additionally, the monitoring is often recorded, so the doctor can examine your rhythm at any time.

The step-down unit is much quieter than the ICU so you should be able to rest better at night. During the day, you will still receive a lot of nursing care—probably more than you want. Nurses will continue to help you do breathing exercises several times a day, take your vital signs every hour or two, and insist that you sit up in a chair or walk several times a day.

If you are a smoker, you will probably be visited by a respiratory therapist two or three times a day. The therapist may perform percussion and vibration—using a heavy-duty vibrator on your chest wall to help free up and clear secretions. You may also receive some breathing treatments. These consist of inhaling an aerosol of bronchodilating (opening the bronchial tubes) medications to help you clear secretions and cough more easily.

You will rapidly learn that the less you cough and the less deeply you breathe, the more attention (often unwanted) you will get from the nurses and respiratory therapists. This is because coughing and deep breathing are critical in preventing pneumonia from developing after surgery. Pulmonary complications are the most common problem to develop between the third and seventh days after surgery, but they can be prevented by coughing and breathing deeply.

You will also be weighed every day, and probably asked to measure your urine output each time you go to the bathroom. Your fluid intake will also be monitored closely and you will be asked to keep a record of everything you drink. It is normal for a person to gain several pounds of water weight during surgery. If your cardiac function is adequate, this will be removed naturally over the first week after surgery. If you are retaining further water, or not losing the water weight fast enough, your doctor may order some tests or prescribe some medications to help remove it. If you "cheat"—for example, have a soft drink without charting it—the doctor may think you are retaining fluid and could order medication unnecessarily.

During this part of your recovery you may notice that your appetite is poor (and the typical hospital food doesn't help). A dietitian will visit you and may suggest supplementing your diet with some high-protein drinks until your appetite returns to normal. The dietitian will also furnish you with information on heart-healthy diets for you to follow both in the hospital and when you go home (see chapter 14).

The period after surgery is the best time to begin changing your eating habits, if you haven't done so already. It is also important for your spouse to meet with the dietitian. Eating healthy works much better if all family members share it. You may truly believe you won't touch the double-fudge ice cream with caramel sauce that your spouse keeps in the freezer, but you probably will eventually.

You will also begin working with physical therapists during this time, although at first it will probably be limited to walking and some range-of-motion exercises for your arms and legs. You will get to know the physical therapists much better in the days to come.

Finally, almost everyone who has bypass surgery suffers through some emotional difficulty during the first week after surgery, and to a lesser extent for the next month or two. When you consider that you have literally had a life-saving procedure performed, this is not surprising. Many people find they have days or hours when they are almost euphoric, followed by days or hours of significant depression. These symptoms will lessen over time, but if they are severe, let your doctor know. A lot of things can be done to ease these symptoms, and no one, especially you, benefits when you try to "tough it out."

The emotional problems may be made a little worse by the changes in medication that occur during this time. For the first day or two after surgery, you received large amounts of narcotics and sedative medications. During your time in the step-down unit and on the hospital floor, the dose of these medications can be reduced significantly. The doctors and nurses are careful to make sure you don't develop physical dependence on these medications, but the changes can be enough to affect your mood to some degree.

The Remainder of Hospital Recovery

Once your doctor has decided you no longer need a monitored bed, you can be transferred to a regular hospital room. In some cases you may go there directly from the ICU without spending time in a step-down unit. In this latter case, your first few days on the floor will be similar to what would happen in the step-down unit, although you won't have a heart monitor attached. Most people, however, will return to the floor about their fourth postoperative day.

The remainder of your hospital stay will consist of allowing the body's natural healing processes to take place and introducing you to the therapies that you will continue for quite a while after you get home. The healing process accelerates from this point forward. Barring any complications, most of the drains and tubes will have been removed by the time you are transferred to the hospital floor. You may still have a single IV for medication purposes, but this will also be removed soon. Generally, you will be eating normally and able to walk for ten to fifteen minutes at a time by the fourth or fifth day after surgery.

Nurses will continue to weigh you every day, but you will probably not have to measure your fluid intake and urine output any longer. You will still be asked to do deep breathing exercises with the spirometer, and a lot of attention will still be focused on the leg that the vein graft was taken from. The most common time to develop respiratory complications or thrombosis of the leg veins is during the period from three to ten days after surgery.

By a week after surgery, you will probably find that the pain in your leg and chest is markedly decreased. You will still want to protect your chest with a pillow when you cough and will need to be a little careful about pushing with your arms, but there is almost no chest pain otherwise. You will be fitted for elastic stockings for your legs, and you can remove the elastic bandages once these have arrived.

The dietitian will continue to visit you during this part of your hospital stay in order to make adjustments to your diet and to try to find foods you like that will be healthy for your heart. The dietitian will also sit down with you to plan your meals for the first month after you get home. If you were a smoker immediately before surgery, someone from a smoking cessation program will probably visit to provide you with tips for quitting.

You will have physical therapy appointments once or twice each day. At this point there are two goals in physical therapy: to help you recover strength and movement following the surgery and to begin a cardio-vascular exercise program to help restore conditioning to your heart. The program will be closely supervised at first, and you may have an EKG performed during or after your first set of exercises to make sure that it is not straining your heart.

Usually you will be allowed to go home ten to fourteen days after the surgery. This can vary depending on a lot of factors: how much heart damage you suffered before surgery, the number of grafts (or valve repairs) that were required, any complications, and the presence of other diseases that could delay your recovery. If you don't live in the same city the surgery was performed in, the surgeon may ask you to stay in a local hotel for a few more days so that you can continue outpatient therapy.

Continuing Recovery at Home

When you return home, you will have to take it easy for several weeks. You probably will see the surgeon about ten days after you are discharged, and again about three weeks later. You will also return to see your cardiologist two to four weeks after surgery. Usually the cardiologist will be the person who continues to care for you over the long term and will handle your heart medications from this point forward.

One restriction you will have for at least six weeks after surgery is that you are not to drive. Many people feel perfectly capable of driving within a few weeks after arriving home and resent this restriction. It is important that you not drive, for several reasons. The motions of steering a car put pressure across the sternum and could delay healing of the breastbone. Additionally, a sudden, sharp pain from an incision could cause you to jerk the steering wheel and cause an accident. Most importantly, though, if you did have an accident, the force of your chest hitting the steering wheel could cause severe injury, since the breastbone is not yet healed and does not provide its normal protection to the heart. For the same reason, your surgeon may recommend you not wear the shoulder part of the lap-shoulder seatbelt while riding in a car during the first six weeks after surgery.

Because the veins remaining in your leg are not used to carrying all the leg's blood flow, you should not stand without walking for prolonged periods (more than thirty minutes) during the first month after surgery. After this time you can stand for whatever period is comfortable, as long as it does not cause swelling in your leg. Your surgeon may also ask you to elevate your leg for an hour or so once or twice a day. When elevating your leg, you should put it in a position such that the knee is bent slightly, since this will maximize the ability of the veins to remove blood from your leg's circulation.

By six weeks after surgery, many people have resumed all their usual activities. For others, the recovery period may take longer, but virtually everyone is back to normal by three months after surgery. Most people who wish to do so can return to work within three months.

A few long-term complications sometimes occur after open-heart surgery, and you should be aware of them. The most worrisome involves infection in one of the incisions. If you begin to run a low-grade fever, or if an area of an incision becomes swollen, red, or drains fluid, you should call your doctor immediately. Treatment of surgical infections must be started immediately in order to avoid long-term complications.

Occasionally a nerve inside the chest or near the incision in your leg becomes trapped in scar tissue from the incisions. The pain from a trapped nerve has several characteristics different from the usual post-operative pain. Nerve pain tends to have a shooting or shocking character, is associated with movement, and may radiate down the leg or across the chest. It does not respond well to pain medication. If you have symptoms like this, make sure you mention them to your surgeon during your return visit. Effective treatments are available.

Long-Term Recovery

During the first six weeks to three months after your surgery, you will probably go to physical therapy about three times a week (some people will go daily for the first month). During this period, the therapy will begin to concentrate more on cardiovascular conditioning rather than recovery from surgery. Records will be kept of your progress, and as the therapy progresses, you will be asked to do more exercises on your own at home. Once therapy has ended, you should be able to continue your exercise program entirely on your own at home.

The benefits of this exercise program cannot be overemphasized, especially for people with coronary artery disease. Cardiovascular conditioning will dramatically improve the amount of activity you can do without having symptoms. It will also help you lose weight and lower the levels of "bad" cholesterol in your blood. It has been shown that people who exercise regularly after surgery are less than half as likely to have another heart attack as those who don't exercise.

It is not sufficient to just "get into shape" and then stop exercising. Those people who complete a postoperative fitness program and then stop exercising lose all the benefit they've gained within three to six months. After this period, they are just as likely to have another heart attack as someone who never exercised at all. Their cholesterol levels will return to pre-exercise levels within two to three months, and they will often regain all the weight they lost.

In addition to exercise, coronary patients should be making major dietary changes while they are recovering from surgery, unless they had already done so. This doesn't necessarily mean you have to lose weight (although that may be recommended). You do, however, need to eliminate cholesterol and saturated fats from your diet. The hospital dietitian will have started you on a heart-healthy diet, and other sections of this book cover diet in more detail. Proper diet alone can decrease the risk of future heart attacks by at least 25 percent.

Neither exercise nor diet is as important as stopping smoking, however. In fact, if you continue to smoke, you will negate much of the benefit of diet and exercise programs. People who have a heart attack or bypass graft and continue to smoke are two to three times more likely to suffer a new heart attack than those who quit smoking.

Almost half of the people who have bypass surgery do not follow these recommendations, feeling that now they have a new set of coronary arteries, they don't have to worry about their heart disease anymore. It is vitally important to remember that neither coronary bypass surgery nor angioplasty has been shown to prolong the life expectancy of a person with coronary artery disease. Symptoms are reduced dramatically and the person can live a more normal life, but life expectancy is no greater than that of a person with similar heart disease who did not have surgery.

It has been shown in many studies, however, that exercise, proper diet, and stopping smoking each can prolong the life of a person with coronary artery disease. It is clear that how you take care of yourself following surgery is more important than the outcome of the surgery itself.

Chapter 11

PACEMAKERS AND ARRHYTHMIA CONTROL

At times, rhythm disturbances of the heart (see chapter 6) become so severe that a pacemaker is required to restore a normal heartbeat. Pacemakers may be inserted temporarily for patients who are suffering severe arrhythmias following a heart attack or cardiac surgery, or permanently for persons having long-term problems with cardiac rhythm. In very rare situations, an implanted defibrillator may be surgically placed in patients who have lethal dysrhythmias. In a few other situations, surgery may be performed to destroy a focus of abnormal beats or an abnormal conducting path.

In general, dysrhythmias require treatment when they cause significant symptoms: fainting or passing out, shortness of breath, or heart failure. Treatment will also be required if the dysrhythmia is of a type known to be associated with ventricular fibrillation or sudden death.

In most cases, permanent pacemakers and surgical procedures are used only when medical therapy and the normal healing process have failed to restore a functioning rhythm to the heart. In some cases, such as people who develop third-degree heart block, doctors know from experience that the problem will not be treatable unless a pacemaker is inserted.

How Does a Pacemaker Work?

Pacemakers are electronic devices that put out a sudden burst of electrical current at regular intervals. The current is carried through wires, called the pacemaker leads, that are inserted into the heart tissue itself. When the small electrical current reaches the heart tissue, it initiates a contraction of the heart muscle, similar to the one that should occur with a normal heartbeat. Although the current is enough to cause the heart to contract, it is far too small for the patient to feel.

The pacemaker itself is a device about 2½ inches in diameter and less than ½ inch thick, enclosed in a waterproof metal casing that is usually made from titanium. Most of the space inside the pacemaker is taken up by an advanced type of battery that usually lasts from three to ten years before it needs to be replaced. The remainder of the pacemaker contains microcomputer chips and electronic circuitry. The pacemaker lead consists of a single cord containing several wires, insulated by silicone rubber or polyurethane.

Pacemakers are marvelous examples of miniaturization technology. Years ago, they simply contained a single circuit, called a pulse generator, that sent out an electronic impulse every second. Most modern pacemakers contain several other circuits and advancements. The pulse-generating circuit can be programmed to send out impulses at various rates, so that it can be customized to beat at the rate that is best for your heart. There is also a two-way programming circuit that can send and receive signals to and from a computer outside the heart. This allows doctors to change the rate or other aspects of the pacemaker by remote control, and also to receive information from the pacemaker, such as how much energy is left in the battery.

Most pacemakers used today also contain a sensing circuit that monitors the heart's electrical activity. Pacemakers with this capability are called on-demand pacemakers. If they sense the heart is beating adequately, they simply stand by and do nothing. Whenever they sense that the heartbeat has slowed or paused, they begin sending out impulses to "pace" the heart to a faster rate. This has several advantages: The heart and pacemaker won't send out conflicting impulses, the heart can contract normally whenever the sinoatrial node is functioning, and the battery life of the pacemaker is extended, since it doesn't have to send impulses all the time.

Another type of pacemaker, the dual-chamber pacemaker, is used for persons with complete heart block. These people have normal contractions of their atria, but the impulse doesn't reach the ventricles. A dual-chamber pacemaker has a sensing lead in the atria, which senses whenever the atria contract. It then sends an immediate impulse to the pacing lead in the ventricles, providing a coordinated contraction between the atria and ventricles, just as a normal heartbeat would. This prevents the atria and ventricles from contracting simultaneously, which would interfere with the ventricles' filling with blood. Dual-chamber pacemakers also sense when the atrial heart rate speeds up, and automatically increase the ventricular rate to match it. This provides increased blood flow to the body when it is needed, such as during exercise.

Finally, some of the most advanced devices are rate-responsive pacemakers. These are used for some people who don't have a functioning sinoatrial node. These types of pacemakers sense other factors in the body to determine if there is a need for increased blood flow, such as exercise, and increase the heart rate accordingly. One type of rate-responsive pacemaker senses motion of the body, such as would be caused by walking or some other form of exercise. Another senses the rate and depth of breathing and adjusts the heart rate as respirations increase. In either case, whenever the pacemaker senses exercise, it increases the heart rate, providing more blood flow to the body.

The Insertion Procedure and Aftercare

The implantation of a permanent pacemaker is a minor surgical procedure that is almost always performed under local anesthesia in about an hour, usually on an outpatient basis. You should not eat or drink anything for six hours before the procedure. Immediately before the procedure, an IV will be placed in your arm, and you will usually receive a mild sedative.

After arriving in the operating room, you will be connected to several monitors, including an EKG and blood pressure cuff. An area under your collarbone will be shaved and washed with soap containing iodine, and sterile drapes will be placed around this area. Your arms may be loosely strapped to boards along the operating table so that you won't move them if you doze off during the procedure (most people do fall asleep once the procedure has started). The drapes will block your vision of the actual procedure, but someone will remain near your head to talk to you and tell you what is happening.

The doctor will use a local anesthetic to numb the area under your collarbone and will wait a few seconds for it to take effect. You will not feel any pain when the incision is made, but there may be a tugging sensation as the doctor makes a small pocket to receive the pacemaker. This is generally not very uncomfortable. The doctor then inserts a needle into the large vein under your collarbone and threads the pacemaker lead through the vein and vena cava into the right ventricle. An X-ray machine is used to visualize the lead as it is inserted so that the doctor can tell when it is in the proper position.

Once the wires are in position, the doctor will connect them to a temporary pacemaker and a computer. These are controlled by a technician at one side of the operating table, and there will generally be a lot of cryptic conversation between the technician and the doctor as the leads are tested. Depending on the test results, the doctor may relocate the leads to obtain the best possible pacing for your heart.

Once the leads are properly positioned and tested, they are connected to the permanent pacemaker and tested again. Once this testing has proved everything works satisfactorily, it will take the doctor about fifteen minutes to place the pacemaker in the pocket and sew up the incision. The incision will be closed with subcutaneous (under the skin) stitches that dissolve, so you won't have to have stitches removed. Just before you leave the operating room, the entire pacemaker system will be tested again to make certain everything is working properly.

You may spend thirty minutes or so in the recovery room after the procedure, or you may be taken directly back to your hospital room. Usually you will stay in the hospital overnight so that the pacemaker's function can be monitored, but this is not always necessary. You will have a little swelling and pain around the pacemaker incision, but this is quite mild. The swelling will go down in about a week, although there will still be a small bulge in the area from the pacemaker.

You can eat as soon as you feel like it and can shower forty-eight hours after the procedure. Most doctors advise you not to drive or perform vigorous activity with the arm on the side of the pacemaker for two weeks or so after the procedure. This is to assure that the pacemaker lead does not become dislodged from its proper location. After several weeks, scar tissue forms around the lead and anchors it in place. Once this has occurred you can do almost anything you did before the pacemaker insertion. Often you can be more active than you were before.

A few precautions should be taken when you have a pacemaker. You should not shoot a rifle or shotgun from the shoulder the pacemaker is implanted in. (If you hunt, make sure you tell your doctor this *before* the procedure.) You also should avoid strong electromagnetic fields. Pacemaker wearers should generally not have MRI scans and should not work around construction-type electromagnets. Airport monitoring devices and microwave ovens are not a problem for modern pacemakers, however.

The doctor will check your pacemaker every two weeks for a month or so, then every three to six months. The pacemaker battery will eventually need to be replaced, but this may not occur for ten years. A computer-driven magnetic device is used to monitor and adjust your pacemaker when needed. Some of these devices can even be used to give a report to the doctor over the telephone. Once the monitor reports the battery is weakening, you will be scheduled for a replacement. The battery will still have several months of power remaining when it begins to weaken, however, so this is not an emergency.

Temporary Pacemakers

Temporary pacemakers can be inserted if irregular beats occur after a heart attack or surgical procedure but are expected to resolve with time, or if a life-threatening dysrhythmia must be corrected immediately. The leads for a temporary pacemaker are inserted into the large vein under your collarbone via a needle puncture. No incision is needed. The leads are then connected to a boxlike pacing device that remains attached to a stand or the side of your bed. If a temporary pacemaker is needed, it will usually be left in place for several days. At that time it will either be discontinued or a permanent pacemaker will be inserted.

Implanted Defibrillators

Some dysrhythmia problems do not prevent the heart from contracting properly, but rather cause episodes of severe abnormal beats. Usually severe rhythm abnormalities involve ventricular tachycardia, or even ventricular fibrillation. These episodes can result in sudden cardiac death if they are not treated immediately.

When such dysrhythmias occur in a patient who is being monitored in the hospital, external defibrillation is used to try to restore the heart to a normal rhythm. External defibrillators are large boxlike devices attached to paddles that deliver a large jolt of electric current to the chest. A large shock of electricity must be delivered in order for enough current to pass through the chest to shock the heart. Occasionally, defibrillation is used electively to try to restore normal rhythm to a person in atrial fibrillation, a process called cardioversion.

People who have recurrent episodes of ventricular tachycardia or fibrillation that is resistant to medical treatment are at very high risk of sudden cardiac death. In recent years, implanted internal defibrillators have been developed to provide an automatic treatment of such rhythms.

Like pacemakers, internal defibrillators consist of an internal battery, electronic circuitry that senses the heart's electrical activity, and electronic pulse generation circuitry attached to the heart via electrodes. There are certain differences, however. An internal defibrillator must deliver a much larger current than that used by a pacemaker, and the device is correspondingly larger—a bit bigger than a deck of cards.

A more complex set of leads is also required. One set is inserted through a vein like a pacemaker lead to sense the heart's activity. Another set, used to deliver the defibrillating current, is attached to the outside of the heart, or may be inserted in the chest cavity near the heart. Some types of internal defibrillators also have pacemaker circuitry built in, and have the ability to act as both pacemaker and defibrillator.

Because these devices are larger and more complex than pacemakers, they are usually inserted under general anesthesia. The defibrillator itself is usually implanted beneath the skin and muscle of the upper abdomen. A second incision may be required to attach the defibrillating electrodes that go to the heart, and one or two small "tunneling" incisions may be required to pass the sensing/pacing electrode from the vein under the collarbone to the defibrillator.

Because the procedure is more complicated, and because the condition being treated is more lethal, most people will be admitted to the intensive care unit for monitoring after this surgery, even though they will feel well and be alert. Usually the patient remains in the ICU for twenty-four hours and remains in the hospital for several days. As with pacemakers, the device will be programmed and fine-tuned using a computer-driven device during the first several days after implantation.

Once the defibrillator senses an abnormal beat, it will try to pace the heart back to a normal rhythm. If this is not successful, or if the device senses ventricular fibrillation, it will deliver a defibrillating shock through the electrodes around the heart. If you are conscious when this happens, you may feel a thump or jolt in the chest.

The defibrillator keeps an internal record of how often it is required to pace the heart or deliver a defibrillating shock. The doctor will probably check this information every two weeks until he or she feels assured it is working as well as possible. After that time, the doctor will still want to monitor you every one to three months.

These devices have been shown to reduce dramatically the incidence of sudden cardiac death in persons who have lethal types of dysrhythmia. They do not prevent the dysrhythmia from beginning, however, and most people will get light-headed or even faint when the dysrhythmia occurs. For this reason, persons with implanted defibrillators should not drive cars or operate dangerous equipment until they have been cleared to do so by their doctor.

Surgery for Dysrhythmias

Very few dysrhythmias benefit from surgical treatment. There are two types of exceptions, however. Wolff-Parkinson-White syndrome is a congenital condition in which people are born with an accessory conducting path between the sinoatrial node and the atrioventricular node. They are predisposed to have episodes of rapid heart rhythms that can be very dangerous. The other exceptions are people who have abnormal pacemakers that are localized to a very specific part of the heart tissue.

In either case, if medical treatment is not successful, surgical or cardiac catheterization procedures may be indicated. Catheter ablation (elimination) procedures are performed during cardiac catheterization (see chapter 7). Special electrical studies are used to determine exactly where the accessory pathway is in patients with Wolff-Parkinson-White syndrome. Once the pathway is carefully mapped out, the doctor inserts a special catheter with a needlelike tip into the pathway. Radiofrequency energy (similar to microwaves) is used to heat the tip of the catheter, burning the accessory pathway until it is destroyed.

In some cases the accessory pathway's location is not accessible to a catheter. In these situations, open-heart surgery is required to allow a surgeon to cut through the pathway. Surgery, of course, carries more risks than catheter ablation and is reserved for those cases when it is absolutely necessary or when ablation has failed to correct the problem. Open-heart surgery may also be required to remove an abnormal pacemaker that is localized to a specific bit of heart tissue. The procedure is quite successful but is rarely needed.

Section III

WHAT YOU CAN DO YOURSELF

Chapter 12

CARDIAC RISK FACTORS AND WHAT YOU CAN DO ABOUT THEM

Risk Factors

What Are Risk Factors?

Everyone has heard about cardiac risk factors. Unfortunately, a lot of the "facts" we hear are actually advertising concerned with selling "healthy" products, not all of which are actually healthy. Another frequent source of information is poorly researched or written articles ("Garlic Diet Prevents Heart Disease" is always popular) in certain magazines and television shows. Neither source tends to give a lot of solid information.

Few people have a thorough understanding of what "risk factor" means. A lot of people believe that if you have a risk factor present, you will develop the disease. Others think that if you eliminate the risk factor, you won't get the disease. Neither is true. Cardiac risk factors are simply conditions known to be associated with developing heart disease, especially coronary artery disease. If you have high cholesterol levels, for example, you are more likely than others to develop coronary disease, but you are not certain to develop it. If you lower your cholesterol you are less likely to develop it, but there is no guarantee you won't.

There is also a lot of misunderstanding about what things are risk factors. Everyone knows that smoking, lack of exercise, and high-cholesterol diets are bad for the heart. Most people, however, would be hard-pressed to name three other risk factors. Even fewer people understand which risk factors can truly be changed or how much benefit the change can have.

In this chapter we will discuss the modifiable risk factors—things that you can change significantly. Nonmodifiable risk factors—things that can be changed not at all or to only a slight degree—will be covered in less detail.

The four most common modifiable risk factors are: smoking, obesity (or bad diet), lack of exercise, and emotional stress. Most people can readily identify the first three as cardiac risk factors. Emotional stress is less closely linked to heart disease, but most authorities feel it plays a role in developing heart disease, at least in some people.

Nonmodifiable risk factors include genetic inheritance, gender, and the presence of other diseases. The genes you were born with cannot be changed, but in some cases the conditions they cause can be treated medically. For this reason a few genetic conditions are considered somewhat modifiable. Some people, for example, have a genetic condition that causes very high cholesterol or triglyceride levels and results in the early development of atherosclerosis and coronary disease. Medication can't change the presence of the condition, but it can lower the cholesterol levels, reducing the risk to some degree.

Gender cannot be modified (at least as far as the heart is concerned), and until the age of menopause women are at much less risk for developing heart disease than men are. After menopause women lose the protective effect of estrogen and suffer heart disease at a rate similar to men. Supplemental estrogen therapy may slow or reduce the effects of estrogen loss, however, so while gender is not modifiable, loss of estrogen is.

Likewise, diseases that increase the risk of developing heart disease may not be modifiable, but medical treatment may minimize their effects on the heart. Hypertension is an excellent example of a modifiable disease. If hypertension is properly treated, the hypertensive person's risk of heart disease is only slightly higher than that of people who have never had hypertension. On the other hand, diabetes also predisposes a person to heart disease, and while control of diabetes may reduce the risk of heart disease slightly, even well-treated diabetics are more likely to have heart attacks than are other individuals.

How Do Risk Factors Cause Heart Disease?

We certainly don't know all the things the various risk factors do that cause heart disease. Many of the risk factors for coronary artery disease cause an increase in a person's risk for developing atherosclerosis, often by increasing levels of fats in the blood. In general, high blood levels of triglycerides (fats) and total cholesterol are associated with an increased rate of atherosclerosis.

Since fats don't mix with water, they are found in the blood only in association with protein molecules. The fat-protein molecule combination is called a lipoprotein. Low-density lipoprotein, or LDL, carries most of the cholesterol found in the blood. It is often referred to as "bad" cholesterol, since it is LDL that furnishes the cholesterol that enters atherosclerotic plaques. High-density lipoprotein, or HDL, carries less of the total cholesterol in the blood. HDL is often referred to as "good" cholesterol, because it carries cholesterol away from the blood vessels to the liver for removal. Doctors sometimes refer to a third type of lipoprotein called very-low-density lipoprotein, or VLDL. This lipoprotein carries triglycerides, which are discussed below.

About one-third of the cholesterol found in the bloodstream comes from the diet. The remainder is comprised of cholesterol the body itself has manufactured for various purposes. Several risk factors can elevate the level of LDL: diets high in cholesterol, lack of exercise, smoking, genetic conditions that result in the body manufacturing too much cholesterol, or genetic conditions that prevent the body from removing cholesterol efficiently. Obviously, when these many risk factors affect the levels of LDL in the blood, we cannot say that the presence of any one will definitely cause a heart attack.

Smoking increases the risk of heart disease in many different ways. Smoking not only increases the level of LDL, it also reduces the level of HDL. Even those smokers whose LDL levels remain low are at increased risk of developing atherosclerosis, although we are not certain why. Smoking also increases the workload of the heart while reducing its blood and oxygen supply. People who have a heart attack or bypass graft and continue to smoke are two to three times more likely to suffer a new heart attack than are those who quit smoking.

Risk factors can affect the heart in other ways. Genetic problems can directly result in valvular defects of the heart or congenitally abnormal arteries that alter the normal circulation. Hypertension increases the amount of work the heart must do, and it also enlarges the heart, which compromises its blood supply. Lung and kidney diseases can also increase the heart's workload. Excess weight is associated with high levels of LDL, but it also places further strain on the heart and increases the likelihood of hypertension and diabetes.

For some risk factors, we cannot determine exactly what they do that increases the risk of heart disease—we simply know that they do increase the risk. Diabetics, for example, are much more likely to develop coronary artery disease than are other people, because they are more likely to develop sclerosis (closing off) of their arteries. There is a lot of argument as to why they develop arteriosclerosis, however.

How Much Difference Can Controlling Risk Factors Make?

We have known since the 1960s that a diet low in cholesterol and saturated fat can reduce the level of LDL in the bloodstream. Normal people who simply make these changes in their diet can expect a reduction of 10 percent or more in their cholesterol levels. For people with very high cholesterol levels, diet and an anticholesterol drug can reduce blood cholesterol levels by about 20 percent. Other studies have shown that for each 1 percent drop in cholesterol, the risk of having a heart attack during the next five years drops 2 percent. A 20 percent drop in cholesterol, therefore, could result in a 40 percent drop in the risk of heart attack.

The Coronary Drug Project study in the 1970s studied men who were known to have coronary heart disease. Those who were treated with a drug to lower cholesterol levels had 20 percent fewer heart attacks than the control group which did not receive the drug. A similar study of a different drug performed in Sweden in the 1980s showed a 34 percent decrease in the incidence of heart attacks for those patients whose cholesterol levels were lowered. In fact, nine of eleven major studies during the last three decades showed that coronary heart disease patients who lowered their LDL levels had significantly fewer new heart attacks than those whose levels remained high or borderline.

Other studies have shown that the atherosclerotic plaques blocking the coronary arteries will continue to progress in more than half of people who do not make lifestyle changes. The vast majority of people who change their diet, quit smoking, and exercise will have no further increase in the degree of blockage. In some people (about one out of six), diet and exercise will actually shrink the plaques.

Smokers are twice as likely as nonsmokers to have heart attacks, and those who continue to smoke after a heart attack are twice as likely to have a second attack. People who quit smoking, however, will reduce their risk of future heart attacks. Three years after a person stops smoking, they are at no higher risk of heart attack than are people who have never smoked.

For other risk factors, the statistics are not as clear and not as well studied. It is certain, however, that people who actively reduce the risk factors that can be modified have a much lower incidence of developing heart disease. Those who already have heart disease can reduce the risk of their disease worsening. While many doctors don't like to quote statistics (although they do like to argue about them), almost all agree that control of risk factors can reduce the chance of future heart attacks by at least one-half.

It is important to remember that risk factors are not simply additive, but rather they multiply each other. A person who has two risk factors—for example, a smoker who also never exercises—is not twice as likely to develop heart disease as a person without risk factors; he or she is 3 or 4 times as likely. A person with four risk factors may be 12 or 15 times more likely to develop heart disease than a person with no risk factors.

Smoking

The Risk of Smoking

Smoking is a very high-risk habit, resulting in a markedly increased rate of not only cardiac and vascular disease, but also of several types of cancer, emphysema, and other disorders. According to the Surgeon General, 20 percent of all deaths in the United States are the result of diseases caused by cigarette smoking. Smoking directly causes about half million deaths per year in the United States—more than AIDS, drug abuse (including alcohol abuse and drunk driving), and all accidents combined.

Smokers in general are at least twice as likely as others to develop coronary artery disease. The risk is proportional to the amount smoked and the duration of smoking. People who smoke heavily (two packs per day or more) are at least three times as likely to develop coronary disease. The risk is also proportional to the number of years smoked: someone who has smoked for twenty years is twice as likely to have heart disease as someone who has smoked for ten years. The risk of smoking continues in those who have suffered a heart attack. Those who continue to smoke are about twice as likely to have a second heart attack as those who quit.

No one is absolutely certain what substances in cigarette smoke are most harmful, since normal smoke contains over four thousand different chemicals that are absorbed by the body. We do know that something in tobacco smoke increases the amount of LDL in the blood and decreases the amount of HDL, resulting in a higher risk of atherosclerosis. Smoking also increases the blood's tendency to form clots over atherosclerotic plaques, raising the risk of heart attack and stroke. There is evidence that some chemical in tobacco smoke also damages the lining of blood vessels, making clots even more likely to occur.

Other substances in smoke cause changes in the blood circulation and in the heart itself. Nicotine increases both blood pressure and heart rate. This combined effect dramatically increases the amount of work the heart must do, while at the same time reducing the amount of blood flowing to the heart itself. Smoke also contains carbon monoxide, which reduces the blood's ability to carry oxygen. This means the body's tissues require more blood circulation each minute in order to receive the oxygen they need. The heart must therefore pump even more blood, while at the same time receiving blood that contains less oxygen.

Nicotine and carbon monoxide also cause the arteries to constrict. If a diseased coronary artery constricts too much, its diameter may narrow until it can't deliver blood to the heart, causing an episode of angina. If the constriction lasts too long, a heart attack can result. The same changes that affect the heart can affect the other blood vessels of the body. That is why smokers are much more likely to develop peripheral vascular disease or abdominal aortic aneurysms than are nonsmokers.

Smoking low-tar and low-nicotine cigarettes does decrease the risk of lung cancer for smokers but does not seem to reduce the incidence of heart disease. Many studies suggest this is because people smoking low-nicotine cigarettes actually smoke more frequently and inhale more deeply. As a result they receive as much nicotine and may actually receive more of the other chemicals contained in smoke.

Smoking also blunts the effect of healthy activities. Many of the benefits that would result from exercise and healthy eating are lessened if the person continues to smoke. Smoking is especially dangerous for people who have other risk factors, such as diabetes or a strong family history of heart disease. These individuals may be at four or five times greater risk than those who have the same risk factor but don't smoke.

The number of people smoking in the United States has decreased. At one time, almost half of all Americans smoked, but this rate has dropped to about 30 percent currently. It is expected to drop to 25 percent by the end of the century. Unfortunately, the message does not seem to be reaching young people. The only group that currently has an increasing rate of smoking is young females.

The Risk of Secondhand Smoke

Although controversy continues about how harmful secondhand smoke is, most studies show that it has some association with heart disease and cancer. It is known that the risk from secondhand smoke is proportional to the amount inhaled. It is impossible to determine exactly how much secondhand smoke a person inhales, so it is impossible to quantitate the risk precisely. Certainly, avoiding very smoky areas and insisting that people not smoke in your home are reasonable ways to help avoid secondhand smoke.

What Happens When You Quit Smoking?

We all know the risk of heart disease is reduced when a person quits smoking. A person who smokes is twice as likely to die from heart disease as a nonsmoker. If that person quits smoking the risk is reduced to 1.3 times that of a nonsmoker. Even older people who have smoked for many years benefit. For example, a fifty-year-old who has smoked for thirty years will reduce his risk of dying during the next fifteen years by 50 percent, and his risk of having a heart attack during that time by 30 percent if he quits.

Stopping smoking is certainly the most important thing any heart patient can do to help prevent further heart attacks. The benefits of quitting smoking begin almost immediately but are not maximized for about two years after quitting. Carbon monoxide levels in the blood begin to drop within a few days of quitting, and within thirty days are almost undetectable. The pulse rate slows and blood pressure usually drops slightly by about the same time.

Many smokers are surprised to find they actually cough a bit more right after they quit. This is because cigarette smoke actually suppresses the cough reflex. (Not having a cigarette all night is one cause of the morning "smoker's cough.") The cough experienced after you quit smoking is actually the body ridding itself of the smoke particles that have built up in the lungs. Most people who quit smoking find that the cough goes away in two or three months. At about the same time, they usually sense that breathing is easier and they are less short of breath with exertion.

Improvement in lung function continues for the next six months, as does an increase in HDL and a drop of LDL in the bloodstream. A few years after quitting, an ex-smoker will have reached the maximum benefit and is only slightly more at risk to develop heart disease than is a person who has never smoked.

Nicotine Withdrawal

Another thing that happens when you quit smoking is withdrawal symptoms. Nicotine (and perhaps some of the other chemicals in smoke) is a drug that affects many organs in the body, including the brain. Over time, the brain develops a dependence on nicotine; it is used to the chemical's presence and its function is altered for a while when the drug is removed. Withdrawal symptoms usually begin within a few hours after quitting smoking and peak several days later.

Some people (it seems ex-smokers are sometimes the worst offenders) minimize the withdrawal symptoms or believe they aren't real. There is no question that withdrawal from nicotine is real. It is no coincidence that the success rate of people who try to quit smoking is about the same as people who try to stop a heroin or cocaine addiction. Between 75 and 90 percent return to the drug after any single attempt at quitting. Don't let the number dismay you, though. Most people who really want to quit are eventually successful, although it may take several attempts.

The most noticeable symptom of nicotine withdrawal is a craving for cigarettes. Other common symptoms include restlessness and sometimes difficulty sleeping, anxiety, and irritability. Headache, difficulty concentrating, and sometimes mild depression are also reported. The major symptoms last a week to two weeks, but they may return as periods of "secondary withdrawal" for several months. Secondary withdrawal symptoms usually last only a few hours, or at most a day. The episodes of secondary withdrawal become shorter and less frequent with time and usually disappear within a few months of quitting. The symptoms can be reduced, although not eliminated entirely, by nicotine replacement therapy such as nicotine gum or skin patches.

A psychological component acts in concert with nicotine withdrawal. Smoking is a habit, often of many years' duration. It is not surprising that people have difficulty finding something to do with their hands, or have a strong desire for a cigarette after certain activities. Like all habits, this one is difficult to break, and the physical withdrawal symptoms make it more difficult.

Finally, almost everyone who thinks about quitting smoking is concerned about weight gain. Most ex-smokers will experience a few pounds of weight gain during the first two months after quitting, and about one-third of them will gain 5 pounds or more. This occurs partly because nicotine has some mild appetite-suppressing effects and partly because some people use snacking as a replacement for the hand-to-mouth activities they previously associated with smoking.

For the great majority of people who quit smoking, any weight gain is temporary. Only 10 percent of smokers who quit will be heavier after one year than they were before they quit. From a heart health standpoint, the minor cardiac risk of even a significant weight gain is more than offset by the huge reduction in risk that occurs when you stop smoking.

Methods to Help Stop Smoking

A lot of things can be done to help you quit smoking. In fact, entire books and seminar series are devoted to that topic. There is no way to cover all that material here, and it is strongly suggested that you investigate some of these other sources for further help (see appendix E).

The most important thing that leads to a successful attempt to stop smoking is to approach it with the seriousness it deserves. Simply announcing you are quitting and putting the cigarettes down has a very low success rate. After several such unsuccessful attempts, people often become depressed and feel that quitting is hopeless.

It is important to enlist the help and support of people around you as you attempt to quit. The key words are *support* and *attempt.* Telling others you are quitting can provide further incentive to stop, and also helps you avoid temptation if the others are smokers. While it is important for family and friends to understand that you are trying to stop, it is also important that they realize it is not helpful to nag a person in nicotine withdrawal. If you relapse back to smoking, they should encourage you to try again, but telling you how disappointed they are in you will probably just increase your desire to smoke. It is important to remember that the average smoker makes three or four attempts to quit before being successful.

Quitting cold turkey—that is, giving up cigarettes suddenly and tolerating the withdrawal symptoms until they pass—is successful for a lot of people. Many others find that they are unable to tolerate the withdrawal symptoms without some other forms of help. Nicotine replacement therapy, support groups, hypnosis, and a variety of stop-smoking programs have all had success. There is no single easy way to quit, however. None of these techniques is much more successful than any other. Using several at once is probably better than using just one.

Nicotine Replacement

Nicotine replacement therapy is available as chewing gum or skin patches. Replacement therapy gives you a dose of nicotine similar to what you would get from smoking and thus eliminates the physical withdrawal symptoms during the period of breaking the habit of smoking. The idea is that it is easier to deal with the physical dependence and the psychological habit one at a time.

Each form of therapy has its advantages. The gum can be used as needed, mimicking the intermittent doses of nicotine that a person would get from smoking. The major disadvantage of gum is that the dose is not very well regulated. Chewing the gum vigorously can deliver very high levels of nicotine. Some people also find that the gum irritates the inside of their mouth.

Theoretically, one would use less and less gum as time goes on, but this doesn't always happen. Nevertheless, almost every doctor would agree that the pure nicotine delivered from gum is less harmful than the four thousand chemicals delivered by cigarette smoke.

Nicotine patches have the advantage of delivering an accurate, constant level of nicotine to the bloodstream. They also are available in various strengths, allowing a well-regulated tapering of the dose. Some smokers find that the steady level of nicotine delivered by the patches does not stop their withdrawal as well as the variable levels supplied by nicotine gum, however. It also takes several hours for the patch to start delivering a steady dose of nicotine after it is applied, so there may be some withdrawal symptoms during patch changeovers.

It has been demonstrated that smokers who use nicotine replacement therapy have a slightly higher success rate when they quit than those who go cold turkey. Nicotine replacement is not a guarantee of success by any means, however, and will certainly not be successful in a person who is not motivated to stop.

Support Groups

There are many types of smoking cessation groups. Some are run by insurance companies or hospitals and are free or low cost. Others are for-profit groups that charge a significant fee. Most groups base their program on instruction of techniques that help people quit more successfully, techniques to help cope with withdrawal, and some form of mutual support. Many of the programs combine stress management alternatives, nicotine replacement therapy, and exercise. Others emphasize mutual support groups. Knowing other smokers are quitting with you and feeling the same way you are can help decrease the cravings and increase your motivation to quit.

The success rates with such groups are usually higher than those experienced by smokers trying to quit by themselves. None of them have long-term success rates of even 50 percent, however, and no reputable program will make such a claim. Any group that charges a large fee and promises spectacular success rates should be viewed with suspicion.

Other Professional Help

Many people have reported that hypnosis and posthypnotic suggestion have helped them to quit smoking. Most hypnotherapists feel that repeated sessions over at least several weeks, if not several months, are required for success. Because there is a great deal of individual variation in both the therapist's techniques and the patient's suggestibility, it is difficult to determine how successful hypnotherapy is.

Other techniques that have been used as an aid in quitting smoking include acupuncture, diet, and herbal remedies. Scientifically, none of these techniques has been rigorously tested, and some of the claims made for them appear patently false. Nevertheless, any therapy that helps you to quit smoking is beneficial, and none of them does anything that would be considered harmful.

Weight and Diet

Obesity

Most people realize they are a little bit overweight, but few consider themselves to be obese (see also chapter 14). Medically speaking, however, almost 75 percent of Americans are obese, and 10 percent are "morbidly" obese, meaning their obesity is so severe that they are at high risk of early death. There are complex formulas and measurements for calculating what constitutes obesity, but standard height-weight ta-

Table 12-1: Height-Weight Guidelines for People over Age Thirty-Five

This table provides a rough estimate of weight ratios for each inch of height. Generally, men of a given height should weigh in the upper half of the range, while women should weigh in the lower half.

Height (inches)	Acceptable Weight Range (pounds)
60	108–138
61	111–143
62	115–148
63	119–152
64	122–157
65	126–162
66	130–167
67	134–172
68	138–178
69	142–183
70	146–188
71	151–194
72	155–199
73	159–205
74	164–210
75	168–216
76	173–222
77	177–228

Data adapted from Dietary Guidelines for Americans, *U.S. Department of Health and Human Services, 1990.*

bles are usually sufficient to give us a good idea of whether we are overweight (Table 12-1).

Those who are more than 10 percent above the maximum weight recommended for their height are considered to be obese. Their risk of dying younger than their normal life expectancy is about 1.1 times that of the general population. Those who are 50 percent over their ideal weight are considered morbidly obese. Their risk of dying is more than double that of nonobese people. If a person becomes even more over-weight, the risk of early death skyrockets. People who weigh twice their ideal weight are twelve times more likely to die young than are people who are not obese.

Obesity itself is not a major risk factor for heart disease. It does, how-ever, place a significant strain on the heart as it attempts to pump blood through all that extra tissue. One estimate is that each 2 pounds of ex-cess fat adds almost a mile of capillaries through which the heart must pump blood.

More importantly, obesity tends to cause other cardiac risk factors to be elevated. Obese people are twice as likely as nonobese people to have high cholesterol. They are three times as likely to have high blood pres-sure and diabetes. They are also likely to have blood clots in their veins, which can lead to pulmonary embolism. If obese people require surgery or invasive procedures such as heart catheterization, they are four times as likely to develop complications.

Correcting obesity requires more than going on a diet. Lifestyle changes including diet and exercise are necessary to take weight off and keep it off. Most experts agree that it is better to not diet at all than to yo-yo—for example, taking off 20 pounds over six months and then putting it back on over the next six.

A word about diet medications: Many of the newer combinations of medications have shown dramatic weight-loss results. It is not at all clear, however, that people using these medications keep off the weight. Medications may seem to be the easy way to lose weight, but most physicians are skeptical that weight loss alone has much benefit for heart patients unless they change what they eat and improve their level of exercise. For this reason, most doctors do not recommend diet med-ications for cardiac patients.

The exceptions are patients who are morbidly obese. For them, weight loss is one of the highest priorities. Even so, heart patients should always consult a cardiologist before taking any diet medications. Some of them have profound effects on the heart, and others can interact with cardiac medications.

Dietary Cholesterol and Saturated Fat

Improving their eating habits is one of the easiest changes most heart patients can make to benefit their health. Everybody is aware that foods high in cholesterol and saturated fat are bad for the heart, but few realize how much of a difference eating right can make to cardiac risk factors.

As mentioned earlier, about one-third of cholesterol in the bloodstream comes from the diet. Also important are the triglycerides, the fats that we eat. Fats are generally classified as saturated (the carbon atoms are all attached to other molecules) or unsaturated (two or more of the carbon atoms are not attached to any other atoms). Almost all fats contain a mixture of saturated, monounsaturated (unsaturated at one location), and polyunsaturated (unsaturated at several locations) molecules, but the proportion of each differs depending on the source of the fat. Once in the body, some of the saturated fat is converted into cholesterol, and for this reason all heart-healthy diets recommend limiting saturated fats.

The typical American diet contains huge amounts of fat—more than one-third of all the calories we eat. Almost half of this is saturated fat. We also eat a large amount of cholesterol, about 440 milligrams per day on average, which is far more than people in most other countries consume.

All the cholesterol we eat comes from animal products. Meat, poultry, eggs, milk, and fish contain significant amounts of cholesterol. Some amount of fat is contained in almost every type of food, although fresh fruits and vegetables have very low levels. Meat, milk, and eggs contain large amounts of saturated fat, as do some vegetable oils (coconut and palm oil, especially). Corn and safflower oils, on the other hand, contain mostly unsaturated fat.

Dietary changes can make a huge difference in serum cholesterol and triglyceride levels. It is especially important to recognize that total cholesterol intake, saturated fat intake, and total fat intake all have an effect on the blood cholesterol levels and the proportions of LDL and HDL in the blood. Additionally, total calorie intake will directly affect weight loss or gain.

Dietary recommendations will vary for each person, but they are usually based on the need to lose weight and the levels of cholesterol and triglyceride found on the serum lipid profile (see Table 14-1). All coronary artery patients should make as many positive changes in diet as practical, however, even if their lipid profiles are not in the undesirable range. Specifically, a diet for a person with heart disease should be similar to that described as a "moderate cholesterol reduction" diet, while persons with elevated lipid profiles should consider a "strict cholesterol reduction" diet (see Table 14-2).

Eating foods that contain water-soluble fiber (such as oat bran) also lowers the blood cholesterol level. One study showed that men eating 100 grams of water-soluble fiber a day had a decrease in cholesterol levels of almost 20 percent. Others have shown smaller, but still significant, decreases in cholesterol levels.

Generally, a heart-healthy diet will begin to lower blood cholesterol levels within two to three weeks. The higher the blood cholesterol level is to begin with, the greater the reduction that can be expected. Most Americans can easily obtain about a 10 percent reduction in serum cholesterol from diet alone. Since the risk of future heart attack is reduced twice as much as the percent reduction in cholesterol, diet alone can result in a 20 percent reduction in heart attack risk.

Sodium Intake

Salt intake is not an issue for people with some forms of heart disease, but it is extremely important for those with congestive heart failure or high blood pressure. Salt causes the body to retain fluid, which worsens the swelling experienced by congestive heart failure patients. More importantly, the fluid can overload the heart, worsening the heart failure.

For hypertensive patients, reducing salt intake alone can be effective in reducing blood pressure. Salt also works against some of the medications used to treat high blood pressure. Since the average American consumes twice as much salt as is recommended, it is probably a good idea for everyone to lower their salt intake.

Lack of Exercise

A sedentary lifestyle—one with very little exercise—markedly increases the risk of coronary artery disease (see also chapter 13). The Framingham heart study, a study that followed several thousand people for many years to determine the various factors that were risks for heart disease, showed that inactive people are five times more likely to have a heart attack than are those who exercise regularly and are much more likely to have a stroke.

Lack of exercise causes both direct and indirect cardiac risks. The direct risk is weakening of the heart muscle itself, making it a less efficient pump with less efficient circulation. The indirect risks are increases in the levels of LDL in the bloodstream and increases in the chance of the individual developing hypertension or obesity.

Persons who exercise have lower blood levels of LDL (bad) cholesterol and lipids, while HDL (good) cholesterol levels are increased. When people who have inactive lifestyles begin to exercise, they show an increase in their HDL cholesterol and a decrease in their total cholesterol. Exercise may be especially beneficial to postmenopausal women. Women who exercise regularly after menopause have much lower total cholesterol and higher HDL levels than women who don't exercise.

Another benefit of exercise is weight control. Exercise not only increases the number of calories burned off during the day, but there is evidence that people who exercise regularly have decreased appetite. The benefit of exercise for weight control is therefore twofold: It increases the number of calories used while at the same time decreasing the appetite. While some people can successfully diet without exercising, they are the exception rather than the norm. Often, people who diet only for weight control simply "yo-yo" back and forth in weight, a situation most doctors feel is worse than simply staying obese. People who both diet and exercise are much more likely to keep weight off.

Exercise also has the benefit of allowing people to perform more physical activity with less effort. People with heart disease who exercise, especially those with coronary artery disease, are more able to perform normal activities without having symptoms of their disease interfere. The benefits of exercise are every bit as true for older people as for younger people. In fact, the Framingham heart study showed that people between the ages of fifty-five and sixty-four were as likely to benefit from exercise as those in their thirties and forties.

People who don't exercise are more likely to develop high blood pressure than are people who do exercise. Exercise can also reduce the severity of high blood pressure. Studies have shown that people with mild to moderate hypertension (diastolic blood pressure 90 to 100) require less medication once they start an exercise program.

Stress and the Type A Personality

It is extremely difficult to study the effects of stress on heart disease (see also chapter 15). For one thing, it is difficult to define stress. One person may find working two jobs very stressful, while another may find that work is relaxing. It is also difficult to separate the direct effects that stress causes on the body (it changes the levels of certain hormones and other chemicals) from the secondary effects. For example, people who have what are generally considered high-stress lifestyles are more likely to smoke and overeat and less likely to exercise. Additionally, different people have different physical responses to stress. Some people can exist comfortably in what would generally be considered a very high-stress lifestyle. Others find that they become physically ill with what would seem to be mild amounts of stress. To some degree, at least, this physical reaction to stress is just that—physical. No amount of mental toughness can keep a person from developing an ulcer, for example.

The effect of stress on heart disease first began getting attention in the 1960s, when researchers described what they called the "type A personality." The type A personality is usually defined as competitive, hurried, and driven to achieve. The original research focused on males in the 1960s, so type A personalities were generally considered to be "workaholics" who focused entirely on their jobs. It has become clear, however, that type A people are not always workaholic. There are plenty of type A housewives and volunteer workers.

Type B people, on the other hand, tend to be relaxed and unhurried. They are less focused on achievement and goals and tend to accept their current situation. Most studies agree that type A people are about twice as likely to have coronary disease as are type B people. It is not clear whether this difference is directly related to personality type or is related to the higher number of risk factors that go along with a type A lifestyle. Current opinions tend to give more weight to the associated risk factors than to the personality type itself.

It is clear, however, that some people with coronary artery disease and some other heart diseases have more symptoms during times of high stress and are a little more likely to have a heart attack during such periods. Stress causes physical changes in the body that can increase the workload of the heart.

During periods of stress the body releases several chemical transmitters that cause changes in the circulation: adrenaline (also known as epinephrine), noradrenaline, and several types of cortisone. Adrenaline and noradrenaline have the most direct effects on the heart. Both chemicals increase the heart rate and raise the blood pressure, two things that dramatically increase the heart's workload while decreasing its blood supply.

You've experienced the results of these chemicals any time you've been really frightened—for example, if you've barely avoided having a car wreck. You probably felt your heart pounding rapidly in your chest, and you may have had a slight tremor, become suddenly sweaty, or felt nauseated. All these effects are caused by adrenaline and noradrenaline.

This response varies from individual to individual. Some people are so-called hot reactors. Such people have dramatic physical responses to stress, with much more severe increases in heart rate and blood pressure than others. You may know such persons—they are often the ones who become red-faced and tremble when they are angry.

It is less clear whether chronic stress can actually cause heart disease. There is evidence from large studies that people who have chronic stress are slightly more likely to develop coronary artery disease and high blood pressure than are less stressed people with similar cardiac risk factors. The problem with interpreting these studies is that they must arbitrarily define what stress is. For example, most studies define working more than fifty hours per week as stressful, but for some people this is not true.

It seems more clear that people with a solid social support network have a lower incidence of heart disease than people who do not have close friends and relatives. Married people, in general, are at a lower risk of heart disease than single people and tend to live longer. Some studies suggest that people who live in the same city as their family of origin, and those who feel that they have several close friends, are also less likely to develop heart problems.

While the stress link to heart disease is not absolutely certain, most doctors recommend that those people who have heart disease or are at high risk of developing it take measures to minimize stress in their lives. Much evidence suggests (but does not prove) that people with high-stress lifestyles will lower their cardiac risk if they make changes to minimize stress.

Stress and Depression Caused by Heart Disease

Whatever effect stress has in causing heart disease, it is obvious that people feel a lot of stress when they find out that they (or a loved one) have heart disease. Fear of the effects of the disease, concern about the financial and lifestyle changes that could occur, and fear of dying or becoming incapacitated can be almost overwhelming, especially at first.

It is very common for patients and family members to experience mild to moderate depression following a heart attack or heart surgery. Often these symptoms are subtle and are more likely to be recognized by a family member or friend than by the affected person. Moodiness, lack of energy, loss of appetite, and altered sleep patterns are common symptoms of depression. In some cases the symptoms are more severe, especially in the period of recovery between 30 and 120 days following a heart attack or surgery.

There are two important facts to realize concerning such depression: It is usually temporary, and it can be treated. Most patients and spouses report that their mood and feelings have returned to normal within three or four months. This is even more likely when the patient takes an active role in the recovery process. Making lifestyle changes to reduce the risk of future heart attack seems to have a beneficial effect on depression.

Some people have more severe or long-lasting depression. These people often benefit from taking antidepressant medication, participating in a cardiac support group, or both. Support groups are often organized in the same centers where patients go for exercise and physical therapy. It is important that a cardiologist be consulted before antidepressant medications are started, however. A few of these medications can have adverse effects on the heart.

The role of tranquilizers and sleeping pills for treating anxiety and depression is more controversial. Most physicians feel they are useful on a temporary basis. Most also believe they can be useful if used occasionally during periods of increased stress. When taken regularly on a long-term basis (several months or more), however, tranquilizers and sleeping pills tend to increase depressed feelings. The potential for physical dependence also arises when any tranquilizer or sleeping pill is taken for a long period.

Estrogens, Gender, and Menopause

The Protective Effect of Estrogen

Most people are aware that men are more likely than women to have heart attacks. This difference is especially pronounced during middle age. The risk of heart attack for men begins as early as age thirty-fvie and is significant by age forty-five. The risk for women does not become significant until well after menopause.

Heart disease is still the leading cause of death in women, however, and 47 percent of all heart attacks occur in women. The major difference between the sexes is that women, on average, begin having heart attacks about ten years later in life than men. This is because the female hormone estrogen has a protective effect against developing atherosclerosis and coronary artery disease.

It is the presence of estrogen, not simply a lack of testosterone (a male hormone), that is responsible for the protective effect. Estrogen is known to raise levels of HDL in the bloodstream and lower levels of LDL. After menopause, the levels of estrogen drop dramatically and atherosclerosis may begin. Within ten years following menopause, women develop atherosclerosis at a rate equal to men. By age sixty-five, there is no difference in heart disease rates between men and women.

It is noteworthy that women who smoke increase their heart disease rate even more than male smokers. Smoking seems to eliminate much of the protective effect of estrogen, even as it causes the other effects known to increase the rate of heart disease.

In June 1990, the Food and Drug Administration's Fertility and Maternal Health Drugs Advisory Committee concluded that estrogen replacement therapy may reduce a woman's risk of diseases of the heart and blood vessels. Postmenopausal estrogen replacement seems to restore some (but not all) of the protective effect that women have before menopause. Most studies show that heart attack risk is reduced about 30 percent if estrogen supplements are taken.

These supplements appear to increase the risk of uterine and possibly breast cancer, however, so their use must be weighed on an individual basis. It is also unclear how much estrogen a woman must take to gain this protective effect. Female smokers probably should not take supplemental estrogen for cardiac reasons, since they are at higher risk of cancer and stand to benefit much less from the cardiac protective effect.

Gender Bias in Heart Disease

For many years the vast majority of research on heart disease has been performed on men. There were several reason for this: Coronary artery disease was generally considered a male disease; it was often easier to get males to participate in research studies; and drug companies did not want to use women of childbearing age in any drug studies because of the potential liability of birth defects.

There is a widespread popular belief that women have fewer heart attacks than men or die from heart disease less frequently. Even though this belief is basically false, it has been shown to affect not only the general population, but also physicians. A report in 1987 showed that, given similar symptoms of chest pain, doctors were six times more likely to order cardiac catheterization if the patient was male than if the patient was female. Men are also more likely than women to undergo coronary angioplasty or coronary artery bypass surgery.

There is some debate concerning how much of this effect is bias on the part of physicians and how much simply represents women's lower risk of coronary disease. Other studies have suggested that if the symptoms are truly similar, women are just as likely as men to undergo invasive testing and surgical procedures.

No one is certain, however, whether there is a difference between the symptoms experienced by men and by women. It may be that women with similarly severe coronary disease have fewer symptoms than men do. The National Institute of Health has commissioned several long-term studies to clarify this topic, but they will not be completed for several more years.

In the meantime, it is possible that women may need to take a more active or insistent role in the diagnosis and treatment of their heart disease. This may mean getting a second opinion if a woman feels that she has not been thoroughly diagnosed or sufficiently treated. It may also mean that a woman should be sure to inform her doctor of any significant change in symptoms.

Diabetes and Other Diseases

Diabetes Mellitus

Diabetes mellitus is a disease (or possibly a group of related diseases) in which the body does not regulate its supplies of sugar properly. The liver converts much of the food we eat into glucose, a type of sugar that the cells can readily use for energy. The hormone insulin, which is manufactured in the pancreas, allows the cells to take up glucose and use it for energy. Another hormone, glucagon, causes the liver to increase the blood's sugar level.

Type I diabetes (also known as childhood or juvenile diabetes or insulin-dependent diabetes) occurs when the pancreas cannot manufacture insulin to enable the cells to take up glucose properly. Type II diabetes (also known as adult-onset or noninsulin-dependent diabetes) is a result of the cells not responding properly to insulin, although insulin is present.

Type I diabetes affects about one million Americans. Since they have very low insulin levels, they must take supplemental insulin injections to avoid hyperglycemia (too much glucose in the blood). Hyperglycemia can cause coma and a host of other severe complications. Even taking insulin properly is not a total solution for Type I diabetes, however. The most complicated injection regimens can still fail to provide the continuous levels of insulin that the body would automatically make in response to eating and physical activity. As a result, even a well-controlled Type I diabetic patient usually has glucose levels that are often lower or higher than normal.

Type II diabetes is much more common than Type I, affecting about ten million American adults, many of whom are not aware of their condition. It tends to occur much more frequently in people who are overweight and in those with a family history of diabetes. Because the pancreas still makes insulin, the symptoms are not as severe as those of Type I diabetes, and fewer Type II diabetics need to take insulin. Diet, weight loss, and oral medication are often sufficient to control this form of diabetes.

People with either type of diabetes are very likely to develop vascular disease, as well as other complications. Since the coronary arteries are a common site of diabetic vascular disease, many diabetics develop coronary artery disease and have heart attacks. Since diabetes also interferes with the protective effect of estrogen, its effect on the heart is more significant for women than for men. Men with diabetes are twice as likely as other men to have coronary artery disease, while women with diabetes are five times more likely than other women to develop coronary disease.

For many years, a debate has raged among physicians concerning whether keeping "tight control" of blood sugar (meaning that levels are kept very near normal) can help lower the incidence of heart disease for diabetics. The debate continues. Most physicians believe that tight control is theoretically beneficial, but many feel that it is not possible to maintain tight enough control to actually reduce the risk of coronary disease. All agree that diabetics who have very poor control—for example, those who frequently forget their medication or who eat too much—are at higher risk.

Regular exercise may increase insulin sensitivity, improving blood glucose levels and helping control Type II diabetes. Adult-onset or non-insulin-dependent diabetes is also less likely to develop in people who exercise regularly than in inactive people.

Lung Disease

Chronic obstructive pulmonary disease, or emphysema, is frequently the end result of years of smoking. Persons with the disease are also likely to have developed coronary artery disease—not because of the emphysema itself, but because the heavy smoking that causes such lung damage is likely to result in atherosclerosis as well.

Emphysema and some other lung diseases distort and destroy many of the capillaries that make up the pulmonary circulation. As a result, pulmonary hypertension—high blood pressure in the pulmonary arteries—can develop. This has the same effect on the right side of the heart that hypertension has on the left side: the chambers dilate (balloon outward) and the cardiac muscle tissue hypertrophies (thickens). Eventually, right-sided heart failure can result from such pulmonary disease.

Infections in People with Valvular Heart Disease

Any person with valvular heart disease must take special precautions to avoid bacterial infections. (Viral infections such as colds and flu are not a problem.) A damaged heart valve can serve as a focus for bacteria to grow on. Because of this, any time bacteria enter a patient's bloodstream, there is a high risk of endocarditis, an infection of the interior lining tissue of the heart and its valves.

People with even slight damage to their valves must take antibiotics any time they are even slightly at risk of having bacteria enter their bloodstream. This includes bacterial infections such as sinusitis or strep throat and having dental or minor surgical procedures performed.

Chapter 13

EXERCISE AND PHYSICAL ACTIVITY

Next to diets, probably no health-related activity gets more attention than exercise. Exercise shows fill up cable TV time, exercise equipment is advertised almost everywhere, and opinions about the best type of exercise are like noses—everybody has one and they're all a little different.

Everyone agrees that exercise is beneficial. People who exercise regularly have a lower rate of heart disease, a lower incidence of hypertension, lower blood cholesterol, and less obesity. People who already have heart disease are at least as likely, if not more likely, to benefit from exercise as are other people. They can improve their endurance and reduce the symptoms of heart disease, while at the same time lowering the risk of future problems from heart disease.

However, a heart patient has to approach exercise differently than a thirty-year-old who has gotten a little out of shape. Aerobic exercise, meaning exercise that increases the body's use of oxygen, is the key to improving cardiovascular health. Sudden, brief bursts of exercise, such as weight training or push-ups, are not especially beneficial to the heart and lungs, since they don't increase the body's oxygen requirements over a long period of time. The cardiovascular system benefits most from sustained, repetitive exercise such as brisk walking, bicycling, swimming, or jogging.

The Benefits of Exercise

The amount of physical work your body can do can be determined by measuring the amount of oxygen consumed during maximum exercise. This maximum oxygen uptake reaches a natural peak in the late teens and early twenties and then slowly declines with age. A typical sixty-five-year-old has about 70 percent of the exercise capacity of a twenty-five-year-old. This only represents averages, however. With steady exercise the physical capacity of any individual can be increased.

The benefits of increasing exercise capacity are numerous. A person can walk farther and be more active; fewer symptoms will occur during minimal activities. Shortness of breath and fast heart rates during everyday activities become less frequent. The body becomes more efficient at using insulin so the severity of diabetes is lessened.

Persons with high blood pressure seem especially likely to benefit. Several studies in people with mild to moderate hypertension (diastolic blood pressure 90 to 100) found that exercise was as effective as medication in controlling their high blood pressure. Most hypertensive people who exercise regularly for one year are able to stop or at least reduce their blood pressure medication.

The benefits of exercise are every bit as true for older people as for younger. In fact, the Framingham heart study, a study that followed several thousand people for many years to determine the various factors that were risks for heart disease, showed that people between the ages of fifty-five and sixty-four were every bit as likely to benefit from exercise as those in their thirties and forties. Women are as likely to benefit as men, especially after menopause.

Exercise, Cholesterol, and Atherosclerosis

Many studies have documented the beneficial effect that exercise has on blood cholesterol levels. The blood levels of cholesterol and lipids are decreased in people who exercise, while HDL (good) cholesterol levels are increased, slowing or even halting the progression of atherosclerosis. When people who have inactive lifestyles begin to exercise, they show an increase in their HDL cholesterol and a decrease in their total cholesterol. (This benefit is lessened in people who continue to smoke, however.)

Exercise may be especially beneficial to postmenopausal women. After menopause, levels of HDL decrease while levels of total cholesterol and lipids increase. Women who exercise, however, have lower total cholesterol and higher HDL after menopause.

Exercise and Weight

One of the major benefits of exercise is weight control. Most studies show that the majority of obese people do not eat much more than nonobese people, they simply expend fewer calories because of their inactive lifestyle. Exercise not only increases the number of calories burned off during the day, but there is evidence that persons who exercise regularly have a decrease in appetite. There is a therefore a twofold benefit of exercise on weight control: increased calories used, at the same time as appetite decreases.

In the average person, aerobic exercise burns off 10 calories per minute. While one episode of exercise doesn't use up enough calories to make a big difference in weight, exercising aerobically for thirty minutes four times a week uses up an additional 1,200 calories a week. Done regularly, this would result in the loss of about 1.5 pounds per month.

Trying to diet without exercising actually causes the number of calories used daily to decrease. This is part of the reason that people "stop losing" weight during a diet. Exercise will minimize the decrease in calories burned that occurs with dieting. If exercise decreases your appetite, it can also make dieting easier.

Exercise and Coronary Artery Disease

Most people are aware that lack of exercise is associated with a risk of developing atherosclerosis and coronary artery disease, but they might not be aware of how significant that risk is. The Framingham heart study showed that inactive people are five times more likely to have a heart attack than are those who exercise regularly. It also showed that inactive people are more likely to have strokes.

It is obvious that all the above effects would be beneficial to people who have coronary artery disease, and there are other benefits as well. With exercise, the muscles become more efficient at using oxygen, so the demands on the heart are decreased. The heart itself pumps more efficiently in people who exercise, and some studies suggest it may develop "collateral" circulation (additional blood vessels) with regular exercise. The heart also beats more slowly in a person who is in good physical condition. Since the heart itself receives blood only during the period between contractions, this allows more blood flow to the heart itself.

What Is a Reasonable Exercise Program for People with Heart Disease?

It has been shown that as little as fifteen minutes of aerobic exercise three times a week will have a beneficial effect. To a certain point, the degree of improvement in cholesterol levels, weight, and the other benefits is proportional to the amount of aerobic exercise performed. Most physicians suggest working up to thirty to sixty minutes of aerobic activity four times a week, although some recommend daily exercise.

Medical studies have shown that exercise sufficient to burn 2,000 calories per week provides a significant benefit to people with coronary artery disease. Exercising past this level may provide some additional benefit, but the added benefit is not nearly as great after the 2,000 calorie mark is passed. Table 13-1 shows the amount of calories burned per minute by several common forms of exercise performed by an average 170-pound person and a 130-pound person. Using this example, it is apparent that as little exercise as jogging 200 minutes (about three-and-a-half hours) each week would be sufficient for a 170-pound male to reach the 2,000 calorie per week goal.

It takes some time for many people to condition themselves sufficiently to exercise this much. Most medical literature suggests a period of six to eight weeks for inactive people to build an exercise program to this level. Once a person is conditioned enough to exercise aerobically for thirty minutes three times a week, they will begin to experience benefits. The benefits continue to increase over time. In fact, many studies show that cholesterol levels and blood pressure continue to drop during the first year of an exercise program.

If a person stops exercising, however, the benefits reverse. After six to eight weeks without exercising, most people will begin to show a slow increase in cholesterol and a slow decrease in HDL. Weight gain, increased blood pressure, and increased pulse rate will follow.

Before Starting an Exercise Program

If you have recently been diagnosed with coronary artery disease, or have had a heart attack, your doctor has probably enrolled you in a medically supervised cardiac exercise program already. These programs usually begin two to four weeks after a heart attack, or six to eight weeks after cardiac surgery. The programs usually consist of a few weeks of carefully supervised exercise, with a gradual decrease in supervised exercise and an increase in exercising on your own. Most last three months or so.

Table 13-1: Calories Burned per Minute by Some Common Forms
of Exercise

	230 lbs.	170 lbs.	130 lbs.
Bicycling (13 mph)	14.75	12	9.25
Walking (4 mph)	10.15	8.2	6.25
Jogging (5 mph)	12.6	10.2	7.8
Running (8 mph)	21.9	17.7	13.5
Swimming	18.6	15	11.4
Aerobics (vigorous)	12	10.5	8
Cross-country skiing	21.9	17.7	13.5
Tennis	6.8	5.5	4.2

If you are in such a program, do not make changes without consulting the therapists who are supervising your regimen. Exercise following a heart attack or heart surgery must be monitored carefully. In most cases, the therapists are happy to help you change to a different type of exercise, as long as there is no medical contraindication.

Persons who are not in a supervised program can get as much benefit from starting their own exercise program, provided they take a slow and steady, commonsense approach. *Anyone over age thirty-five who has not exercised regularly during the past year, and any person with known or suspected heart disease should not begin exercising without consulting a physician, however.* Any male over age thirty-five and females over age forty who have a family history of heart disease or known cardiac risk factors should probably have an EKG stress test before beginning an exercise program.

Beginning to Exercise

Most people who have not exercised for a while should begin with walking. Start by walking at a moderate pace until you begin to feel tired or start to feel your breathing increase. Note how long you walked (say fifteen minutes), and continue to walk for this amount of time each day for one or two weeks. If you no longer experience any symptoms with walking for the original amount of time, increase the time five minutes the next week. Generally, you should not increase the amount of walking more than once each week.

Once you can walk briskly for thirty minutes without symptoms, you may wish to try other forms of exercise (although walking is a superb, low-impact exercise). Jogging, bicycle riding, using a stationary bicycle or a rowing or skiing machine are excellent alternatives. Follow the same rules when starting each new exercise. First find out how long you can do it with no shortness of breath and increase the duration or rate of exercise only once a week, or even every two weeks.

With any exercise more strenuous than walking, always add a warm-up and cool-down period. Stretching for ten minutes or so is the best way to warm up. Cool-downs should consist of at least ten minutes of walking, with a couple of two-minute stretching periods. Careful warm-up and cool-down periods (along with moderation) are the best way to minimize muscle soreness after exercise.

As you get in better shape (and after checking with your doctor), you can further increase the intensity of your workouts so that you are slightly out of breath during the period of exercise. Once you have reached this stage, you are truly exercising aerobically. This is the type of exercise that provides maximum benefit for the cardiovascular system. *If you know or suspect you have heart disease, however, you should not exercise to the point of shortness of breath without your doctor's approval.*

Setting Exercise Goals

Few of us have to worry about exercising too much. Most people are more interested in finding out how much exercise is enough. Before worrying about an exercise goal, be certain that you start reasonably as described above. Only after you are taking a brisk walk or jog for thirty minutes four times a week should you even concern yourself with how much to exercise.

One good rule of thumb is the "calories burned per week" concept introduced above. Exercising enough to burn 1,200 extra calories is the minimum needed to gain significant benefits for the heart. Exercising enough to burn 2,000 calories provides excellent cardiac benefit, and although more exercise can help the heart even more, the rate of increasing cardiac benefit slows after 2,000 calories per week is reached. For this reason, most doctors and physical therapists use a goal of about 2,000 calories burned from exercise per week.

As shown in Table 13-1, the amount of calories burned depends to some degree on a person's weight. Smaller people have to exercise more to burn the same number of calories, just as lifting a large weight takes more energy than lifting a small weight. Some exercise specialists feel that you should calculate your calories burned from what you *should weigh,* not what you do *weigh.* This way, you automatically build in some additional calorie burning to help lose weight.

Another method of setting exercise goals is the DIFference plan, for Duration, Intensity, and Frequency. This plan focuses on first reaching a reasonable level of conditioning as described above, and then determining how much to exercise by measuring how hard your heart is working. The pulse rate is usually the best way to measure the amount of work the heart is doing. The maximum rate the heart can attain is fairly constant for people of a given age (see Table 13-2).

Being able to exercise intensely enough so that the heart beats at 70 percent of the attainable maximum rate, and to maintain that rate for thirty minutes, is a goal many cardiologists set for their patients. For example, a fifty-year-old should be able to obtain a heart rate of 170 beats per minute. An exercise program that allows a fifty-year-old per-

Table 13-2: Maximal Heart Rate and the Exercise Target Zone

Age	Max Pulse	Target Zone 70% Max	85% Max
30	194	136	165
35	188	132	160
40	182	128	155
45	176	124	150
50	170	119	145
55	164	115	140
60	158	111	135
65	152	107	130
70	146	102	125

son to exercise with sufficient intensity so that the heart beats at 119 beats per minute for thirty minutes would be an initial goal using the DIFference plan.

With even better conditioning, the goal might be raised to 80 percent or even 85 percent of attainable maximum for age. Most cardiologists recommend simply that you exercise in the target zone of between 70 and 80 percent of attainable heart rate, however. Exercise at this level for thirty to forty-five minutes a day is certainly more than adequate to reap the cardiac benefits of exercise. As discussed earlier, however, most cardiologists think that exercising four days a week is enough to markedly improve a heart patient's condition.

Is There a Downside to Exercising?

Proper exercise is good for everyone, including heart patients. For 90 percent of people with heart disease the problem is actually getting them to exercise. Two other things can be a problem, however—over-exertion and overconfidence.

Overexertion with an Exercise Program

For a lot of people, finding out they have heart disease or suffering a heart attack is a wake-up call. They want to undo the problem caused by years of bad habits or lifelong genetic predisposition, and they want to undo it *right now*. Others remember that they used to jog five miles a day and want to return to that level, forgetting that they haven't jogged in ten years.

Some of the problems of overexertion are minor, such as muscle strain and joint aches. These symptoms can be treated with hot soaks and over-the-counter rubs and liniments. It is important to remember that significant muscle and joint aches are your body's way of telling you you're going to fast. They usually signify that you need to slow down your exercise program for a week or two, and then increase it slowly.

Heart patients, especially coronary patients, need to be careful that they don't exercise to a level that causes them to have angina symptoms or irregular pulse. This is why ALL CORONARY ARTERY DISEASE PATIENTS SHOULD CHECK WITH THEIR DOCTOR EACH TIME THEY INCREASE THEIR LEVEL OF EXERCISE. Often the doctor will want to do a series of stress tests to determine how much the person's exercise level can be increased without stressing the heart. A properly monitored exercise program is safe, but one overdone without supervision can actually trigger a heart attack.

Overconfidence in Exercise

There is an old medical story about a patient who has recently had a heart attack and asks his doctor, "What do I need to change so this doesn't happen again?" The doctor's reply: "Everything." Exercise provides many beneficial effects to heart patients and to otherwise healthy people. It is not a cure-all, however. People who exercise but continue to smoke or overeat do not benefit nearly as much as people who make an entire lifestyle change.

It is not unusual for persons to start an exercise program after a heart attack and begin to feel better and better. Soon they can do more than they could before the heart attack. Often they say "I'm in the best shape of my life." This is true, but too many people then rationalize that being in better shape, they can now smoke safely, eat fatty foods, and return to a high-stress lifestyle.

Even more commonly, they decide that having gotten in good condition, they can now cut down to exercising one or two days a week, which rapidly becomes one or two days a month. As mentioned earlier, the cardiac benefits of exercise disappear within a couple of months of stopping. Another danger is that, feeling better, a person decides not to get that follow-up test the doctor recommended, or to stop taking blood pressure medication. While exercise may indeed benefit a person enough so that medication can be stopped and test results may be negative, this can only be done under proper supervision. And not everyone will benefit to this degree.

Even people without heart problems sometimes falsely believe that sufficient exercise can totally prevent heart problems. Doctors often refer to this as the Jim Fixx syndrome. Fixx, for those of you who don't recognize the name, wrote a series of books on the benefits of running and was himself in superb physical condition. He died suddenly of a massive heart attack.

Exercise is not a substitute for proper medical care and diet. It cannot completely prevent the progression of heart disease and atherosclerosis. It does, however, benefit every heart patient to some degree. It should be looked at as one of several tools you can use to reverse your heart disease, but not the only tool.

Chapter 14

EATING TO HELP YOUR HEART

Improving eating habits is one of the easiest changes most heart patients can make to benefit their health. Entire books are devoted to healthy diets for cardiac patients, including dozens of cookbooks with tasty recipes. With so many groups and individuals touting what is healthy, who should you believe?

Often these people are making a profit from what they sell, so their advice must be viewed with a little skepticism. Furthermore, product labeling is often more of an advertising ploy than a means of giving you real information. Although the government is proposing new regulations, it is simple for a manufacturer to label a new product as "low fat" no matter how much fat it contains. Reading the actual content of fat grams on the back of the package may give you a better idea of what the product actually contains.

It all adds up to confusion for a lot of people. For our purposes, we will discuss the reasons for changing your diet and what types of changes are most appropriate for heart patients. Guidelines showing the fat, saturated fat, and cholesterol contents of various foods are listed in appendices A and B. These can help you make some simple but dramatic adjustments to your food intake. You might also think about investing in a cookbook showing healthier ways to prepare your favorite foods.

Dietary Cholesterol, Fat, and Saturated Fat

What Are They?

Everybody is aware that foods high in cholesterol and saturated fat are bad for the heart, although most people don't really know what cholesterol and saturated fats are. Likewise, most people are uncertain whether unsaturated fats are good, bad, or neutral. To really understand what these various substances are, you need to get an idea of what they are made of and how they are used by the body.

Cholesterol is a waxy substance that the body uses in several ways: It is a building block for many of the hormones the various organs release, it makes up part of the membrane surrounding each of the body's cells, and its breakdown products form part of the bile acids, one type of digestion chemical in the intestines.

The body is fully capable of manufacturing all the cholesterol it needs, but we also eat a lot of substances (basically meats, milk, eggs, and other animal products) that contain cholesterol that the body absorbs and uses. About one-third of the cholesterol in most people's bloodstream comes from what they eat, while the remaining two-thirds is manufactured by the body.

Cholesterol, like all fats, does not dissolve in the water of the bloodstream, so it must be transported through the body attached to protein molecules. As discussed in chapter 12, the two fat-protein molecule combinations that transport cholesterol are low-density lipoprotein (LDL) and high-density lipoprotein (HDL). LDL is commonly called "bad cholesterol" since it carries cholesterol to atherosclerotic plaques in the arteries (as well as other locations). HDL is "good cholesterol" since it carries cholesterol to the liver, where it is broken down and destroyed.

Fats are large molecules that are used by all living organisms to store energy and to make up various membranes within the cells. Fats are often referred to as triglycerides, because they are made up of three long fatty acids attached to a glycerol molecule. All the triglycerides are transported through the body as part of a protein-fat complex called very low-density lipoprotein, or VLDL.

In saturated fats, the carbons atoms are all attached to other molecules. In unsaturated fats, two or more of the carbon atoms are not attached to any other atoms. If the fat is unsaturated at only one location, it is monounsaturated; if it is unsaturated at several locations, it is referred to as polyunsaturated.

Almost all foods contain a mixture of saturated, monounsaturated, and polyunsaturated molecules, but the total amount of fat and the proportion of each type differ in food from different sources. Animal fat tends to contain a lot of saturated fat molecules, while most plant fats are polyunsaturated. The body tends to convert saturated fat into cholesterol, and this is the reason most heart-healthy diets recommend limiting levels of saturated fats. There is some evidence that monounsaturated fats tend to raise the levels of HDL, while polyunsaturated fats have a mixed effect.

Sources

The typical American diet contains huge amounts of fat—about 38 percent of all calories consumed are in the form of fats. Saturated and monounsaturated fats each make up about 45 percent of the fat we eat, with polyunsaturated fat accounting for the other 10 percent. We also eat a large amount of cholesterol, about 440 milligrams per day on average, which is far more than people in most other countries consume.

All our cholesterol intake comes from animal products. Red meat, poultry, and most fish contain significant amounts of cholesterol, as does whole milk. The meats derived from animal organs—brains, liver, kidneys, and sweetbreads—are extremely high in cholesterol. Egg yolks contain probably the highest amount of cholesterol of any food, between 210 and 250 mg in each yolk. Since the goal for most people is to take in less than 300 mg of cholesterol a day, whole eggs must usually be eliminated from the diet. Egg whites, however, are low in cholesterol.

Some amount of fat is contained in almost every type of food, although fresh fruits and vegetables have low levels. The quantity and types of fat varies markedly from food to food, however. Saturated fat is the worst type of fat for patients with heart disease or atherosclerosis, and reducing the amount of saturated fat is a major goal of a heart-healthy diet. In general, beef, pork, poultry, milk, and eggs contain significant amounts of saturated fat. Some vegetable oils contain very little saturated fat, while other types contain huge amounts of saturated fat. Coconut and palm oil, for example, contain more saturated fat than butter or lard. Corn and safflower oils, on the other hand, contain mostly unsaturated fat.

Some saturated fats are worse than others. Three saturated fats in particular have been shown to increase blood cholesterol levels markedly: lauric acid, myristic acid, and palmitic acid. Coconut and palm oil contain high levels of these fats, as does regular butter and the cocoa butter used to make chocolate.

While it is important to avoid all saturated fat, some unsaturated fats are less likely than others to raise cholesterol levels. Linoleic acid, a polyunsaturated fat contained in some margarines and oils, has actually been shown to reduce cholesterol levels. Fish oils, which contain a different type of unsaturated fat, have also been shown to reduce cholesterol levels and to help prevent blood clots from forming. Unfortunately, polyunsaturated fats tend to lower the levels of HDL cholesterol in the blood, which may offset any beneficial effect they have on total cholesterol.

Monounsaturated fats, found in canola or rapeseed-based oils (such as Puritan), can also lower cholesterol levels. Several studies suggest that these oils do not lower HDL cholesterol, but rather selectively lower LDL cholesterol. For this reason, many nutritionists suggest that heart patients use primarily canola and rapeseed oils.

It is important to remember that all fried foods contain a large amount of oil, no matter how carefully they are drained after frying. Potatoes, for example, contain almost no fat, but an order of french fries may contain 30 or more grams of fat—half of an entire day's allotment for most reasonable diets. This is especially important to remember when you eat fried restaurant food, since commercial oils used by restaurants are usually made from palm oil, coconut oil, and animal fats.

The Margarine Controversy

In 1990, a study was released in the *New England Journal of Medicine* claiming that a high intake of "trans" fatty acids, a type of artificially created unsaturated fat, was associated with elevation of LDL and depression of HDL in the blood. Because the artificial trans fatty acids (also known as hydrogenated fats) are a major component of stick type margarines, the idea that "margarine is as bad for the heart as butter" was widely touted in headlines throughout the public press.

Almost every large health organization, including the American Medical Association and the American Institute for Clinical Nutrition, have stated that the research done to date does not demonstrate that margarine is bad for you. Though there is little question that these artificial fatty acids may lower HDL and certainly raise the levels of LDL and cholesterol, it appears that they are no worse in this regard than regular saturated fat such as that found in butter.

In any case, almost all margarine with a high trans fatty acid content is sold in stick form. Tub margarines tend to have low levels of trans fatty acids. Most nutritionists currently recommend that for labeling purposes the trans fatty acid component of margarine should be considered a saturated fat rather than unsaturated.

Dietary Recommendations

Dietary changes can make a huge difference in serum cholesterol and triglyceride levels. It is especially important to recognize that total cholesterol intake, saturated fat intake, and total fat intake all have an effect on blood cholesterol levels and the proportions of LDL and HDL in the blood. Additionally, total calorie intake will directly affect weight loss or gain.

The U.S. Department of Health and Human Services recommends that every heart patient make the following general diet changes:

1. Eat fewer high-fat foods.
2. Especially, eat fewer foods high in saturated fat.
3. Replace part of the saturated fat in your diet with unsaturated fat.
4. Eat fewer high-cholesterol foods.
5. Choose foods high in complex carbohydrates (starch and fiber).
6. Lose weight if you are overweight.

Watching Fat and Calories

Dietary recommendations for each person will vary, but are usually based on the need to lose weight and the levels of cholesterol and triglyceride found on the serum lipid profile (see Table 14-1). People

Table 14-1: Lipid Profile Levels

	Desirable	Borderline	Undesirable
Total Cholesterol	<200	200–239	>240
LDL Cholesterol	<130	130–159	>159
HDL Cholesterol	>45	25–45	<35
Triglycerides	<150	151–249	>249

with coronary artery disease, however, should make as many positive changes in diet as practical, even if their lipid profile is not in the undesirable range. Specifically, a diet for a person with heart disease should be similar to that described in the "moderate cholesterol reduction" diet, while persons with undesirable lipid profiles should consider a "strict cholesterol reduction" diet (see Table 14-2).

Determining the exact number of calories you should consume to maintain or lose weight involves some complicated mathematical formulas based on height, weight, age, and activity level. If you are interested in finding out an exact calorie recommendation, you should probably consult a nutritionist, who can also give you a lot of good dietary recommendations.

As a rule of thumb, however, an average-sized woman will lose weight consuming 1,500 calories per day, while a man will do so consuming about 1,800 calories a day. A more accurate estimate is this: the ideal body weight in pounds multiplied by 12 equals daily calories. If a man should weigh 170 pounds, then his daily calorie intake should be about 170 times 12, or 2,040 calories. If you are overweight, you will slowly lose weight at this intake level. In order to lose weight faster, you can reduce your daily calorie count by another 10 percent, but not more.

To determine how many grams of fat you should consume each day, first determine how many calories you should consume, then multiply

Table 14-2: Moderate and Strict Cholesterol Reduction Diets

	Moderate	Strict
Total Fat (% of calories)	30%	<30%
Saturated	<10%	<7%
Polyunsaturated	10%	10%
Monounsaturated	10–15%	10–15%
Cholesterol Intake	<300 mg/day	<200 mg/day

Total calories will vary depending on body size, activity level, and need to lose weight.

total calories times the percentage of calories that are allowed to be from fat. For example, if your diet is 2,000 calories a day, 30 percent of which should come from fat, you can eat 600 calories from fat a day. Since each gram of fat contains 9 calories, divide 600 by 9 to find out how many fat grams you can consume (66.5 grams in this case). At most, one-third of this (22 grams in the example) can be saturated fat.

Generally, the best way to start lowering fat intake is to start reading labels. Keep a small notebook with columns for calories, saturated fat, and unsaturated fat and jot down what you've eaten. Most food packages list the amounts of calories, fat, and saturated fat for each serving. Be careful to read what the manufacturer considers "one serving" to be, however. For cookies, for example, the manufacturer usually says a serving is one cookie. Your personal serving size may be quite a bit different.

In general, if a label is vague or unclear, stay away from the product. Many manufacturers choose a legal path called "flexi-labeling." Flexi-labeling may say something like, "This product may contain one or more of the following items," followed by a long list of ingredients, most of which are fats. Generally, this means all those fats are present, and the worst fats are present in the largest quantities. If a manufacturer has gone to the expense of minimizing the amount of fat in a product,

Table 14-3: Key Ingredients to Avoid

Any animal fat (including chicken fat)

Chocolate or cocoa butter

Coconut or coconut oil

Egg yolk or egg solids

Hydrogenated fat or oil

Lard

Lauric acid

Mysteric acid

Palm or palm kernel oil

Palmitic acid

Shortening

Vegetable fat*

Vegetable shortening*

Whole-milk solids

Healthy products will list the specific vegetable fats or oils. Products simply labeled "vegetable fat" usually contain palm or coconut oil.

they are proud to proclaim it. Also, watch out for any of the ingredients listed in Table 14-3. All contain large amounts of unsaturated fat.

Several simple changes, taken together, can make a dramatic difference in the amount of fat consumed:

Use only skim or ½ percent milk, and low-fat cheese.

Use only vegetable oil and margarine (canola, corn, safflower, sunflower, or soybean oils).

Avoid hamburgers, hot dogs, luncheon meats, bacon, and organ meats.

Avoid all commercial bakery products (many are amazingly high in fat, but rarely labeled).

Eat meat once a day or less, and limit it to a 6-ounce portion (about twice the size of a deck of cards).

Eat less red meat and more fish and poultry.

Avoid egg yolks (two egg whites can be substituted for one whole egg in recipes).

Trim all fat from meat and all skin from chicken or turkey.

Avoid fatty snacks (chips, nuts, candy bars). Popcorn, baked pretzels, and fruit are good snack choices.

More specific ideas and facts about the fat content of various foods are given in appendices A and B.

Fiber

No discussion about diet can be complete without mentioning fiber. Most of the focus on high-fiber diets in the popular press concerns the cancer-preventing effects of fiber. For heart disease patients, the specific type of fiber eaten is important.

Fiber is categorized as water-soluble if it mixes with water or water-insoluble if it does not. Both types of fiber may lower the risk of colon cancer, but *water-soluble fiber also lowers cholesterol.* It has not been proven exactly how this occurs, but the effect is well documented. One study showed that men eating 100 grams of water-soluble fiber a day had a decrease in cholesterol levels of about 20 percent.

The three major types of water-soluble fiber are oat bran, pectin (found in apples and citrus fruits, and also available as a supplement), and beans. Psyllium, the substance contained in Metamucil, is also a water-soluble fiber. *Wheat bran is not a water-soluble fiber* and has no beneficial effect on cholesterol levels.

Fish Oils

As mentioned earlier, fish oils contain some unique unsaturated fats that are thought to help prevent heart disease. In fact, many health food stores market fish oil capsules as a treatment for coronar ease. While it does appear that fish oil has some beneficial venting atherosclerosis, taking high doses of fish oils can cause several problems.

The amount of fish oil needed to produce the beneficial effect is 30 or 40 grams a day—more fat than should reasonably be consumed as a supplement. Many fish oil supplements also contain a large amount of cholesterol. Finally, fat-soluble pesticides and environmental toxins such as PCB, DDT, and dioxin (which is probably the ingredient in Agent Orange that affected many Vietnam war veterans) are concentrated in fish from many areas, and especially concentrated in the oils from those fish. One study found that 30 percent of commercially available fish oils contained high levels of environmental toxins.

For these reasons, most nutritionists recommend adding fresh fish, especially tuna, to your diet, but not taking concentrated fish oil supplements.

What About Alcohol?

Many studies have demonstrated that one drink of alcohol a day increases the level of HDL cholesterol in the blood. There are conflicting studies about whether this difference actually lowers the risk of heart attack or atherosclerosis, but there is certainly some evidence to support this theory. While few doctors encourage their patients to drink, most now agree that one drink a day may be beneficial. Although anecdotal reports have claimed that certain types of alcoholic drinks—for example, red wine, white wine, or beer—are more beneficial than others, there is no clear evidence to support this contention.

A lot of doctors hesitate to recommend alcohol to heart patients because they fear many patients will decide "if one drink is good, then two will be better." It is clear that significant doses of alcohol (two or more drinks a day) have a direct toxic effect on the muscle cells of the heart.

In fact, alcohol abuse is one of the more common causes of cardiomy-opathy. As is true for so many things, moderation is the key.

How Much Can Diet Reduce the Risk of Heart Attack?

Generally your blood cholesterol level should begin to drop two to three weeks after you start a cholesterol-lowering eating pattern. The higher your blood cholesterol level is to begin with, the greater reduction you can expect. The following several rules of thumb help demonstrate how much you can reduce your heart risk through diet.

1. For every 100 mg of cholesterol eliminated from the daily diet, blood cholesterol should drop 5 mg/dl. Most heart-healthy diets will eliminate between 200 and 300 mg of cholesterol per day (assuming an average pre-diet consumption).
2. Each 1 percent decrease in calories from saturated fat should reduce blood cholesterol about 3 mg/dl. Most heart-healthy diets will reduce the calories from saturated fat about 5 percent.
3. Each 1 percent increase in calories from unsaturated fat should reduce blood cholesterol about 1 mg/dl. Most heart-healthy diets will increase calories from unsaturated fat about 2 percent.

Let's assume that an average person who had a pre-diet cholesterol level of 240 mg/dl sticks to a healthy diet. If this person reached all the goals above, we would expect total cholesterol to drop about 27 mg/dl, to about 213 mg/dl. This is an 11 percent reduction in serum cholesterol from diet alone. Since the risk of future heart attack is reduced twice as much as the percent reduction in cholesterol, we would have achieved a 22 percent reduction in heart attack risk.

Dietary Sodium

Effects on Heart Disease

Salt intake may not be an issue for many people, but it can be extremely important for persons with congestive heart failure and for some people with high blood pressure. The most noticeable effect that salt has on the body is a tendency to retain fluid. This can worsen the amount of swelling people with heart failure experience; more importantly, it can actually overload the heart and worsen heart failure. Salt also works against some diuretic (water-removing) medications that may be used to treat high blood pressure and congestive heart failure.

The average daily American diet contains about 4,000 mg of sodium chloride. Even for healthy persons, the maximum recommended allowance of salt is 2,400 mg, while people with heart disease are usually restricted to 2,000 mg a day. Limiting salt intake means a lot more than simply not heavily salting your food, however.

Reducing Salt Intake

For most people the largest source of dietary sodium is not the salt added at the table, but the salt added to foods during processing. For most people the salt in processed foods makes up about two-thirds of their sodium intake. Canned foods, canned soup, and processed meats often contain a large amount of salt. Read labels carefully. Low-salt foods are usually identified on the front of the label, and the specific amount of salt in each serving is listed. If the label does not show salt content, you should assume that it is high. A single can of condensed soup may contain 1,000 mg of sodium or more.

Salt used for seasoning during home cooking and at the table is the second-largest source of dietary salt. A heaping teaspoon of salt contains 1,500 to 2,000 milligrams of sodium. It often takes some time to get used to cooking and seasoning with less salt, and food may initially taste bland. Most people find, however, that their taste buds will adjust over four to six weeks so that foods taste "normal" again even though they're cooked with less salt. Using more pepper or other spices, or eating more spicy types of food, can make the absence of salt less noticeable.

Be careful with using salt substitutes. Most contain potassium chloride rather than sodium chloride. Large amounts of potassium can be harmful for people with kidney disease. Some diuretic medications interfere with the ability of the kidneys to remove potassium; people taking such diuretics should not add more potassium to their diet. On the other hand, some types of diuretics cause loss of potassium, and a potassium-based salt supplement may actually be helpful.

If you are taking any diuretics, check with your doctor before using a salt substitute, since a buildup of potassium can cause heart irregularities.

Chapter 15

THE ROLE OF STRESS AND EMOTION

For thousands of years, people believed that their emotions literally came from their heart. In modern times, we tend to laugh at this notion, but there may be more than a grain of truth to the idea that emotions affect the heart. As discussed in chapter 12, it is difficult to define what stress is, and even more difficult to determine whether it can cause or worsen heart disease. In the last decade, however, it has become clear that emotional stress and depression do have an effect on patients with heart disease.

Even though we are learning about the effects of certain types of stress on heart disease patients, many people resist making any lifestyle changes in this area. There are several reasons for this. People often think they have no emotional problems and deny that the symptoms of depression or high stress levels apply to them. Even people who realize they are highly stressed often do not want any stress-reducing treatment or therapy, since many feel that admitting to being highly stressed is a form of weakness. Finally, doctors in general (although there are many exceptions) are not nearly as comfortable talking about emotions as they are about atherosclerosis and cholesterol levels.

Nevertheless, heart patients who are interested in doing everything possible to lower their risks must investigate the role that stress and emotions have in worsening heart disease. Many simple techniques can minimize the effects that our emotions have on our hearts.

What Is Stress?

We all react differently to different events in our lives. Psychologists and other mental health professionals agree that no one can predict exactly how a given event will affect a certain person's emotions. They do agree that certain types of events tend to cause a stress reaction in most people. For example, the death of a spouse or child, loss of job or income, moving, serious physical illness, and divorce are all considered to be highly stressful events that affect most people emotionally for months after they occur. Many other life events can cause significant stress for some people but don't affect others.

When a stress reaction occurs, its emotional effects can be documented by certain psychological tests. These reactions not only cause emotional changes, they also cause changes in the physical functions of the body. For our purposes, there is no way to list what events, or how many different events, are required to "stress" a given person. Rather it is much simpler to define stress as whatever causes a person to experience emotional difficulty.

Often, people do not want to admit or talk about the things in their life that cause them stress. In our culture, particularly among males, people often believe that being unable to cope with stress is a sign of emotional weakness. The result is that people who are under stress spend a great deal of emotional energy trying to act as though nothing is wrong, a behavior that usually worsens the physical symptoms of stress.

It is difficult to change the way we react to the situation around us.

It can be even more difficult to change our lives to reduce the amount of stress. Only you can determine whether some situations or emotional patterns in your life require change for your well being. In order to make these decisions, it is important that you understand exactly what effects emotional stress has on your body.

The Physical Effects of Stress

Stress, especially chronic stress (lasting more than three months), affects heart patients physically in two broad ways. The first is through the direct physical effects that stress has on the body. When a person suffers emotional stress, the body releases several chemical transmitters that cause physical changes.

Adrenaline (also known as epinephrine) and noradrenaline are released into the bloodstream shortly after emotional stress begins. These chemicals increase the heart rate and raise the blood pressure, causing a huge increase in the heart's workload and a decrease of the heart's blood supply. You've experienced the results of these chemicals any time you've been badly frightened: your heart pounds rapidly, you may tremble or feel weak in the knees, suddenly start sweating, or become nauseated. All these effects are caused by adrenaline and noradrenaline.

When people are chronically stressed, their levels of adrenaline and noradrenaline remain high, although not nearly as high as after a sudden fright. People who are chronically stressed tend to have a higher heart rate, higher blood pressure, and often a mild resting tremor. They may also have trouble sleeping, another effect of high adrenaline levels.

In addition to adrenaline, people suffering chronic stress tend to have high levels of cortisone in their blood. Cortisone causes several physical effects, including an increase in blood pressure, fluid retention, increased stomach acid (which can contribute to ulcers), worsening of diabetes, and changes in appetite. Several other chemicals in the body are known to be altered by chronic stress, but their potential to affect heart disease directly is unclear.

The second way that stress can affect heart disease is through behaviors that are associated with stress. In particular, there is a strong relationship between high-stress levels and behaviors that can definitely worsen heart disease. Highly stressed people are more likely to smoke, to have unhealthy diets, and to neglect exercise.

The degree of physical change that occurs in the body during stress varies among individuals. Some people are called "hot reactors," because they tend to have a large amount of chemical change in their bodies when they are under stress. Such people may become red-faced and tremble when they are angry. Their dramatic physical responses to stress results in more severe increases in heart rate and blood pressure than other people experience. Even people who are not hot reactors will have significant physical changes when they are stressed.

Do Emotions Really Affect Diseases?

For the last fifteen years, psychological journals have reported numerous studies linking emotions and physical illness. In some cases the links are very logical. We know that stress elevates blood pressure and increases the pumping workload of the heart. It's not surprising then, that psychologists and medical doctors have found that persons with coronary disease are more likely to have angina when they feel stressed.

Other links are less logical, but study after study finds them. Did you know, for example, that numerous studies have found that the emotions of cancer patients predict to some degree how effective chemotherapy will be? Or that people who describe themselves as lonely have a shorter life expectancy than others? While we can't say for certain why emotions could affect such diseases, much evidence suggests that they do.

In psychological studies reported in medical journals beginning in the 1960s, researchers described what they called the "type A personality." The type A personality is usually defined as competitive, hurried, and driven to achieve. Originally, most of the type A personalities identified were hard-driven business and professional men who focused on job success. It has become clear, however, that many housewives and volunteer workers also have type A lifestyles.

Since the original reports, a large number of studies have found that type A people are twice as likely to have coronary artery disease and heart attacks as are type B people. Most of the early studies did not demonstrate clearly whether being a type A person is enough to cause heart disease, or whether the associated behaviors (such as smoking, poor eating, lack of exercise) caused the increased risk. Historically, doctors have given more weight to the associated risk factors than to the personality type. Some recent studies, however, show that even when all the associated risk factors are taken into account, type A people are still more likely to develop coronary artery disease. They are not more likely to develop other forms of heart disease, however.

Similar studies have shown that people who are frequently irritated and angry are much more likely to develop coronary artery disease than people who are more relaxed and tend to "go with the flow." Many different psychological tests claim to define "irritability" or "tendency to anger quickly." No matter which test is used to identify these traits, however, the people identified as "irritable" or "easily angered" on psychological tests almost always have a higher incidence of coronary artery disease.

Not only do stress and anger make a person more likely to develop coronary disease, they can worsen the disease after it has developed. Several studies have shown that people with coronary artery disease have more symptoms of angina during times of high stress and are a little more likely to have a heart attack during such periods. Similarly, people with congestive heart failure are likely to have a worsening of their symptoms during stressful times.

Some studies have demonstrated that people who suffer clinical depression are more likely to develop coronary disease and to have a heart attack. An early 1990s study done at Ochsner Clinic in New Orleans found that depressed patients were more likely to be rehospitalized or to die than nondepressed patients. On a positive note, the study also demonstrated that depressed patients who underwent an extended cardiac rehabilitation program not only lowered their cardiac risk, they also had less severe depression after completing the program.

Perhaps the most important evidence linking emotional stress with heart disease has come from research done in the early 1990s. The Mayo Clinic studied almost 400 people with coronary artery disease who entered a cardiac rehabilitation program. They found that people with high scores on a test measuring psychological distress were 20 percent more likely to have a heart attack during the next two years than were other patients. Psychological distress was actually a stronger predictor of future heart attacks than having diabetes or congestive heart failure.

It has also been shown that people with a solid social support network have a lower incidence of heart disease than people who do not have close friends and relatives. For example, married people are slightly less likely to develop heart disease than single people. Some studies suggest that people who live in the same city as their close relatives are less likely to develop heart problems. Similarly, people who identify themselves as having several close friends and an active social life have fewer heart attacks.

While no one can be certain how strongly stress, anger, and depression are linked to the worsening of heart disease, they obviously have some effect. The link seems closest for persons who have coronary artery disease and are either anxious or angry much of the time. There also seems to be a link between depression and worsening of both coronary disease and congestive heart failure. To date, there are no clear links between emotion and the other forms of heart disease.

Can You Do Anything About Stress and Personality Type?

Many people find it comfortable to believe that the stress level in their lives, and the way they deal with stress, cannot be changed any more than their height or eye color could. "I'm too old to change my ways" or "I was born this way" are the usual responses when such people talk about changing the amount of stress in their life. To some degree this is true. People who are "hot reactors" are always going to have a stronger physical response to stressful events than are "cool reactor" types.

On the other hand, many heart patients have made dramatic changes in their lifestyles and the way that they deal with stress. The first step in making such changes is the same as the first step for changing any other unhealthy behavior: You must be willing to try to change. You must approach stress management the same way you approach diet or smoking, and you must believe that these changes are necessary in order to improve your health.

There are two broad areas where you can make changes. The first is your surroundings (the outside); the second is your own response to those surroundings (the inside). Most people are confused about the responsibility that goes with changing their surroundings. Everyone is willing (even eager) to change the way a spouse, boss, coworkers, or children behave. Unfortunately, these people are rarely willing to cooperate in such efforts, at least not for long. What changing your surroundings really means is changing what (and who) you choose to surround yourself with, not changing the behavior of the people around you.

The first step in changing your surroundings is to recognize what events cause a stress reaction in your body. Notice what things cause you to grit your teeth, feel tension in your shoulders, develop a headache, become irritable, or have trouble sleeping. Other warning signs of stress may be an upset stomach, irritability, or tiredness. Recognize that if you have these symptoms around certain people or events, your body is trying to tell you it is stressed. This concept seems simple, but most of us are so used to ignoring these signs that it takes practice to notice them.

The next step is deciding what changes you can make to alter these situations. Sometimes the only thing you can do is to remove yourself from the situation. After the ordeal of a heart attack, you may be willing to decide you really don't need to keep working in that stressful job, or to continue taking care of your grandchildren five days a week. In other situations, just realizing that you are allowing yourself to react may put things in perspective, and you may decide to forget about some past problems or insults. The twenty-dollar loan your brother-in-law hasn't paid back is probably not worth having an angina attack every time you see him.

Remember, you are the one with heart disease, and you are the one who needs to make these changes. Using your heart disease in an attempt to change the people around you doesn't work because they are not motivated to change. It is appropriate, however, to request someone's help or to refuse to enter into situations that you find stressful. For example, if you constantly find yourself mediating disputes between other people, tell them you find this too stressful and ask them not to involve you in their disputes.

While you can't always change your surroundings, you can change how you deal with stressful situations, or even the everyday events of ordinary life. If you find you feel stressed in certain situations, learn how to avoid them or deal with them in another manner. Many people find that by just concentrating on their own responses, they can talk themselves into a less stressful frame of mind. Driving more slowly, taking something to read when a wait is likely (in the checkout line at the grocery store, for example), and scheduling your day at a slower pace can all be helpful ways to minimize everyday irritations.

Many people find that part of their stress comes from a hectic lifestyle. Organizing what you do and planning ahead can often decrease this type of stress dramatically. Keeping "to do" lists or using a daily planning calendar can do wonders to prevent days with too many scheduled activities. It is important to be reasonable and firm in your planning. Allow plenty of time to drive from one activity to another. Most importantly, learn to say no.

Another important area for change is communication skills. We all know exactly what we mean to say and how we want to say it. Sometimes, however, what others hear from us is entirely different. Some of us frequently find ourselves in arguments because others did not understand what we meant, or did not like the way we said it. We can't change other people's hearing, but we can change the way we communicate.

Two types of communication are likely to lead to frequent misunderstandings and irritation: passive communication and aggressive communication. Passive communicators tend to have trouble saying what they really feel. Often they walk away from a conversation having "bitten their tongue" or feeling like the other person has run over them. Aggressive communicators, on the other hand, often find themselves in arguments that they did not intend to start. They find that other people are often "overly sensitive," and they are surprised to find out that they have hurt someone's feelings or made someone angry.

If you tend to engage in either of these types of communication (and most of us do to some degree), you may want to make a conscious effort to communicate assertively. Assertive communication simply means that you have a right to your opinion, and everyone else has a right to theirs. An assertive communicator says what he or she thinks or feels and then allows the other person to do the same. An assertive communicator says, "We disagree on this point," where an aggressive communicator says, "You don't understand," and a passive person says, "You're probably right." As simple as this sounds, assertive communication tends to avoid angering others, while at the same time preventing you from feeling abused.

Many people find that making some of these simple lifestyle changes dramatically lowers their stress level. Others find that they cannot make many lifestyle or behavior changes; they must focus on the second alternative: changing the way their body responds to stress.

A great first step in changing our reactions to stress is to eliminate the irrational standards that we keep for ourselves and others. "I should be able to handle this," "He shouldn't treat me this way," "I wish I'd been more pleasant"—these are self-destructive messages that we give to ourselves. *Should, would,* and *could* statements generally are ways of saying that things are not acceptable the way they are. They force us to focus on negatives rather than positives.

Changing your internal reactions to stress can be done, but often requires a little outside help. You may find that one or two sessions with a therapist to learn relaxation techniques goes a long way toward lowering the tension you experience during the day. As an alternative, you might join a group to learn some form of meditation, or enter into a support group with other heart patients. Many churches, social groups, and education centers offer stress management classes and self-improvement workshops.

Another alternative is to find a hobby or activity that allows you to relax. Setting aside an hour or two a day to do something you really enjoy can be beneficial. It can be even more helpful if the hobby allows you to join some social groups or meet other people with similar interests.

In some cases, even more steps are indicated. People who suffer severe depression or anxiety may need counseling and medication to help them control their symptoms. Antidepressant medications and tranquilizers may be indicated, at least for a while. It is important to remember that tranquilizers, especially, tend to mask the mental symptoms of stress, but may not change the physical response very much. From the standpoint of heart health, it is much better to make lifestyle and personal changes that actually relieve the stress, rather than to use tranquilizers to mask the symptoms.

Does Lowering Your Stress Level Make a Difference?

Unfortunately, few studies exist to demonstrate whether altering stress levels relieves the symptoms of heart disease. This is largely because it is so difficult to measure whether people have really changed the way they deal with stress. There is some evidence to suggest that stress management helps, however.

Several studies performed in the late 1980s and early 1990s found that heart patients who said that their levels of tiredness and irritability had decreased during rehabilitation were less likely to have a second heart attack than were those who felt no change. Another study found that people who completed a six-week emotional therapy course had a slightly lower mortality rate than those who did not. Three other studies found that coronary patients who participated in any organized activity in order to reduce their stress level were less likely to have a second heart attack than were people who denied they had any need to change emotionally.

Obviously, only you can decide if change is necessary in outside stress or in the way you deal with stress. Be honest with yourself in making this decision. It is perfectly all right to start with some minimal adjustments and perhaps to read a book or two on stress management techniques. If your personal stress level is high, however, getting help by counseling or in a group is much more likely to be beneficial than merely reading about it.

Stress and Depression Caused by Heart Disease

We have seen that stress can contribute to causing heart disease, but it is even more obvious that heart disease causes stress in both patients and their family members. The emotional stress that follows a diagnosis of heart disease tends to be different in the first few weeks than it is a month or two later.

The Initial Response

When a diagnosis of heart disease is made, everyone affected becomes very anxious about how serious the condition is and how it will affect their lives. The fear of dying or becoming incapacitated can be almost overwhelming at first. As these fears decrease, other fears arise about the financial impact the disease can have on earnings and savings, and about the lifestyle changes that may be involved.

During this time, the patient and family members as well may find they are tense and have trouble sleeping. Irritability and forgetfulness are common. Mood swings, ranging from severe depression to euphoria, may occur almost every day. While all this emotional upheaval is occurring, most people feel they should be strong and positive for the sake of their family members.

Talking about these emotions is almost always helpful. Many centers that treat heart disease have counselors or chaplains who talk to patients and close family members. Other centers organize group discussions for heart patients and their families. If these services are not available, just talking to understanding friends, clergy, or other patients in similar situations can help smooth the emotional roller coaster.

If the anxiety or depression becomes severe or seems to be getting worse, be sure to mention these feelings to your doctor. Often, the temporary use of a mild tranquilizer, sleeping aid, or antidepressant can help ease these emotional difficulties. Long-term use of these medications is usually not necessary, and most doctors feel that some form of counseling or therapy should begin if the emotional symptoms remain severe for more than a month or six weeks.

The Delayed Response

During the first weeks after the diagnosis of heart disease or following a heart attack, most people find they are quite busy with tests and therapy. Eventually the recovery phase of treatment slows down, and people begin to readjust to a routine lifestyle. Once this occurs, a significant number of heart patients experience mild to moderate depression.

The symptoms of mild depression are subtle and are more likely to be recognized by a family member or friend than by the affected person. Moodiness, lack of energy, loss of appetite, and altered sleep patterns are common symptoms of early depression. In some cases the symptoms are more severe, and include hopelessness and an inability to enjoy most activities.

This postrecovery depression is usually temporary and can almost always be treated. Most patients and spouses report that their mood and emotions have returned to normal by three to four months following a heart attack or heart surgery. As a general rule, patients who have taken an active role in their treatment, and those who made lifestyle changes to reduce the effects of their disease, suffer less depression and recover from it more rapidly.

If the symptoms of depression are significant, they should be treated. The purpose is not only to benefit the mood of the patient. Heart patients with significant depression have a difficult time motivating themselves to exercise, change their diet, and do the other things necessary to improve their health. Often, treating the underlying depression makes it easier to find the motivation to resume normal activities and participate in therapy.

People who have a more severe or long-lasting depression following a heart attack or other heart problem should see a psychologist or psychiatrist. People with more severe symptoms may benefit from taking antidepressant medication on a long-term basis, or from participating in a cardiac support group or other form of therapy. It is important that a cardiologist be consulted before antidepressant medications are started, however. A few of these medications can have adverse effects on the heart.

The role of tranquilizers and sleeping pills for treating long-term anxiety and depression following a heart attack is controversial. Most physicians feel that these medications are useful on a temporary basis and when used occasionally during periods of increased stress. The long-term use of either tranquilizers or sleeping pills tends to increase depression and can result in physical dependence. Antidepressant medication, however, can be taken safely for years.

Chapter 16

WHAT NEW PROGRESS IS BEING MADE?

The Release of New Technology

Advances in the treatment and prevention of heart disease are occurring at a rapid pace. There is a long delay, however, between the time a new medication or technology is first reported and when it is introduced for general use. Several factors contribute to this delay, none of which is likely to change in the near future. Since you may hear about a new treatment years before it becomes available to you, it may help to understand what takes place after a new technology or medication is announced.

New treatments and technologies are usually first announced as case reports or pilot studies in medical journals or at medical meetings. Basically, a case report means that a doctor has observed a new or interesting phenomenon in a few patients (or sometimes a single patient) and has written a report of these findings. A case report may also describe a new technique or piece of equipment that has been used only a few times. If the report concerns something that might be of benefit to many patients, the reporting doctor or someone else may decide to do a pilot study. This involves trying the new technique in a few cases, usually comparing them to a few other patients who were treated in the standard fashion.

Just because some treatment or medication seems effective in a pilot study, or was reported to work in a few cases, this does not mean it will eventually become widely accepted. In fact, most of the treatments described in such reports are later found to be ineffective or dangerous, and they are abandoned. For this reason, the Food and Drug Administration (FDA) requires that at least one large clinical trial be performed before a new treatment is released for general use.

These large clinical trials often involve hundreds, or even a few thousand, patients. They are usually performed in several medical centers scattered around the country, so that a number of doctors are involved. The FDA monitors these trials to make sure they are done properly and accurate records are kept.

In general, it takes several years to complete such a trial. If questions remain about the effectiveness or safety of the new technique, the FDA may order another trial, resulting in a further delay before the treatment is generally released. After the final trial is complete, it is again reviewed for accuracy by the FDA. The results are then presented to medical groups and published in medical journals.

Most European countries have less stringent testing requirements, particularly with regard to new medications. This is the reason that new medications are often released in Europe several years before they are available in the United States. While most American doctors (and pharmaceutical companies) grumble about the delays of our system, it has some merit. Several medications released in Europe have been withdrawn because of unexpected complications or side effects. This rarely happens in the United States.

After a new medication or technology is approved for general use, other centers publish secondary reports showing the results they obtained using it. Often, these reports show that the treatment is not as effective or has a few more complications than the original trial demonstrated. For this reason, many doctors believe that they cannot have an accurate idea of how effective a new technique or medication really is, or how frequent its complications are, until after it has been in general use two or three years.

This process seems fairly direct, although it is time-consuming. In recent years, however, the introduction of new medical technologies has become complicated by two new trends, both of which seem to be financially motivated. The first trend is the tendency of doctors to release the results of their preliminary tests in the public media rather than through medical journals. In the past, doctors reported new techniques and treatments in peer-reviewed medical journals. In a peer-reviewed journal, other doctors with experience in the field have looked at the report and felt that it was accurate and medically sound.

When preliminary results are released to public media such as newspapers, popular magazines, and television, the study is obviously not peer-reviewed. The reporters will rarely mention that these reports are of preliminary work or that years of further study are required. Instead, they often attach headlines that attract more readers or viewers, such as "New Cure for Heart Disease." The doctor releasing the results gets lots of publicity (which really amounts to free advertising). This publicity also may attract grants for further studies. This is not to say that every doctor releasing a preliminary study to the general press is doing so for financial gain, but it does mean that various motives are involved.

Unfortunately, patients who see such reports often find that the treatment is not available. Or their doctor may refuse to use it in all but the most desperate cases, since it is medically unproven. The doctor's refusal to recommend a newly discovered treatment is generally sound medical advice, following the age-old physician's guideline "First, do no harm." Every doctor is aware of a dozen examples of new treatments that sounded great in an early television report but were later found to be dangerous.

The second trend that affects the introduction of new medical technology is that of managed care. Most health insurance companies, and all health maintenance organizations (HMOs) and preferred provider organizations (PPOs), have personnel to review which treatments are medically accepted for a given condition. Even after a treatment has been studied thoroughly and released for general use, the managed-care reviewers will often label it experimental and refuse to pay for it. In a few states, doctors participating in these groups have signed contracts that prevent them from even discussing treatments that the company has labeled experimental. (Most states are currently moving to make such contracts illegal.)

The legality of an insurance company denying certain forms of treatment is complicated and varies from case to case. During the past decade, many patients have hired attorneys in an attempt to force their health-care provider to pay for a specific treatment. Overall, it appears that less than half of such actions are successful. Even if the legal action is eventually successful, there will be a delay of at least several months before the patient can receive the new treatment.

In many cases, however, the company is not only legally correct but also medically correct in denying a new form of treatment. One or two years after their general release, many new treatments are found to be less effective than older ways of treating the same condition. If, however, an insurance company denies payment for a treatment that has been in general use for three or more years, it is probably appropriate to consult an attorney.

Current Research: Procedures and Devices

It is difficult to determine which technologies and medications now under development are likely to have an impact on the treatment of heart disease in the future. In a few areas, however, so much research is taking place that some new treatment should be released soon. By the time you read this book, several of the technologies listed below are likely to be ready for general release.

Minimally Invasive Cardiac Surgery

Despite numerous technical advances, one aspect of heart disease will be with us for the foreseeable future: some patients inevitably will need surgery. Currently most cardiac surgical procedures require that the patient's breastbone be split lengthwise to allow surgeons access to the heart. At the end of the procedure the breastbone is wired together, and it takes between six weeks and three months to fully heal. Several companies and medical centers are currently testing techniques and devices that will allow doctors to perform open-heart surgery without splitting the breastbone.

Several minimally invasive open-heart surgery techniques are currently being developed by large medical companies and are undergoing clinical tests in medical centers. The techniques use a system of special magnifying lenses and retractors to allow surgeons to operate on the heart through two or three small incisions in the chest. This avoids the need to split the breastbone or to break any ribs. The recovery period after such surgery is dramatically shorter than that following conventional techniques, and doctors believe there will probably be fewer complications.

It is unclear which of the system(s) under development will eventually be released for general use. Some systems avoid the need for heart-lung bypass entirely but can only be used for certain procedures, such as one-vessel coronary bypass grafts. Other systems include the ability to use heart-lung bypass and have been used to perform multiple-vessel coronary bypass grafts and mitral valve replacement.

The initial reports from these procedures have been encouraging. Some persons having bypass surgery with minimally invasive techniques have returned to work less than two weeks after surgery. At the time of this writing (1997) initial FDA testing has been completed on three types of minimally invasive cardiac surgery techniques, and large-scale tests have begun in a few medical centers. It is expected that at least some of these devices will be in general use by the year 2000.

Artificial Hearts and Left Ventricular Assist Devices

Most of us remember the widespread publicity that accompanied the first use of artificial hearts in the 1980s. A few patients had artificial hearts implanted as a temporary measure while they waited for human heart transplants. A few others had animal heart transplants as an alternative to artificial hearts, but this technology has largely been abandoned. All received widespread publicity on television and in newspapers.

To date, a total of ninety-two patients have received the Jarvik-7 artificial heart as a bridge while awaiting heart transplant. Sixty-three of these patients (68 percent) lived long enough to receive heart transplants. Only thirty-five of those patients receiving heart transplants survived (38 percent of the ninety-two original patients), however. Complications of the artificial hearts, especially those involving blood clots and strokes, limit their use to only the most desperate situations.

Left ventricular assist devices (LVADs) are basically mechanical pumps that are used to help the patient's heart pump more effectively. Unlike artificial hearts, left ventricular assist devices are used in addition to the patient's heart, not as a replacement for it. The ventricular assist devices pump a portion of the blood delivered to the left ventricle. These devices differ from the widely used aortic balloon pump (see chapter 9) in that they can be used for several weeks, while the balloon pump is useful for only a few days.

Most currently used LVADs are tethered to large pieces of equipment outside the body, but some newer electrical devices are almost entirely self-contained. A totally implantable ventricular assist device has been developed that is surgically inserted inside the abdomen and connected to the left ventricle and the aorta. Some of the blood arriving at the left ventricle is diverted to the implanted LVAD, which uses an electrically driven pump to force the blood into the aorta.

The pump is connected to a computerized control unit about the size of a deck of cards that is implanted just under the skin. The unit contains an internal rechargeable battery that drives the electrical pump. The internal battery can be recharged by an external coil and battery pack worn by the patient. The external coil can transfer magnetic energy to a second coil in the implanted control device, which converts this energy back to electricity, recharging the internal battery.

When used as a bridge in patients awaiting heart transplants, the ventricular assist device had a post-transplant survival rate of 82 percent, much higher than that of artificial hearts. Unfortunately, the technology required to make such a device safe for long-term use (several months or more) is still many years away.

Cardiomyoplasty

Cardiomyoplasty is an experimental surgical procedure that takes a muscle from the back and uses it in an attempt to help a damaged left ventricle pump more effectively. The procedure was first performed in Paris in 1985 and was repeated a few months later in the United States. It was originally considered a stopgap measure to prolong the life of heart failure patients who were awaiting heart transplant, but it now is being considered as an alternative to transplantation.

Cardiomyoplasty involves repositioning the latissimus dorsi, a large flat muscle from the back, so that one end of it is wrapped completely around a patient's heart. An electrical sensor/stimulator is implanted in the patient's abdomen. It senses the natural heartbeat and sends an electrical impulse to the newly positioned latissimus muscle, causing it to contract with every other heartbeat. The contraction of the latissimus squeezes the heart, forcing blood out of the left ventricle more effectively. The repositioned back muscle requires several weeks of "training" before it is able to help the heart continuously, but after that time it can take over a significant part of the damaged heart muscle's function. The removal of the back muscle causes no deformity or loss of movement, but it does cause a reduction in the strength of the affected shoulder.

The first FDA-approved study of cardiomyoplasty took place between 1991 and 1993 and involved 68 patients. The patients in the study were not bedridden but were extremely limited in their activities. It was expected that about half of them would die within two years without treatment. Twelve months after undergoing the procedure, 70 percent of the patients were still alive, and most showed improved heart function and increased physical activity levels. Many of the patients were able to reduce their doses of heart medication.

At this time, further FDA studies are being undertaken, and the procedure has been performed less than 500 times worldwide. The procedure is now being considered as an alternative to heart transplantation in selected cases. Cardiomyoplasty may be considered in persons with severe heart failure who are not eligible for heart transplantation. The procedure is also less expensive than heart transplantation and eliminates the need to take immune-suppressing medication that is required after transplant.

Because it takes several weeks for the new muscle to be trained and strengthened, patients in the final stages of heart failure are not candidates for cardiomyoplasty. The procedure has a mortality rate of 12 percent during and immediately after surgery; although high, this is not unexpected given the severe condition of those who have undergone it to date. It is premature to predict long-term survival rates for patients receiving cardiomyoplasty.

The current FDA studies will involve 600 patients followed for at least two years; the results should be available by 1999. In the meantime, cardiomyoplasty is being performed more frequently in Europe. If the results of the FDA and European studies are as successful as the preliminary results, the procedure may gain widespread acceptance in the United States by the turn of the century.

Transmyocardial Laser Revascularization

Another procedure, called transmyocardial laser revascularization, may benefit patients with coronary artery disease. The procedure basically involves using a carbon dioxide laser to drill holes through the heart muscle that connect to the cavity of the left ventricle. The theory of the procedure is that oxygenated blood from the left ventricle will flow into heart muscle, carrying oxygen to areas of the muscle that need it.

In a pilot study at the University of Texas in Houston, the procedure was performed on twenty-one patients with severe coronary artery disease who were not candidates for any other type of treatment. Six months after the procedure, fourteen of the patients had a significant decrease in the frequency of angina attacks and an improvement in their exercise tolerance. Five patients had died from heart attacks during the study period, however.

Positron emission tomography (PET) scans, an imaging procedure that can show the biochemical activity and blood flow of the heart muscle, demonstrated that the heart muscle had an increased blood flow after laser revascularization. An autopsy on one patient who died from a heart attack showed that the laser channels were still open and had connected to other parts of the coronary circulation.

Although these results are very preliminary, and they go against some current understandings of the coronary circulation, widespread clinical testing of the procedure began recently. At this time, it is reserved for persons with severe coronary artery disease who have failed, or are not candidates for, coronary bypass surgery.

Artificial Blood Vessels

Currently, coronary artery bypass surgery involves transplanting a vein from another part of the body to replace a diseased coronary artery. This may cause complications in the area from which the vein was removed, and in some people, no acceptable vein is available for transplantation. Artificial replacements for larger arteries, such as the aorta, have been available for many years, but none of these are acceptable as a replacement for coronary arteries because they are likely to cause blood clots.

Several medical research companies are working to develop artificial arteries. Most of these artificial arteries are based on tubes of woven material such as Dacron. Using new technologies, living cells are grown inside the mesh to create a lining almost the same as that of a living artery. Special treatment removes any protein from the cell's surface that might cause a rejection reaction from the recipient's immune system. A different technique takes cells from the recipient before surgery and grows them to line the artificial vessels.

Artificial blood vessels could end the need for using veins in coronary bypass surgery and could allow the surgery to be performed on persons who do not have acceptable veins to use as grafts. This technology is still in animal testing stages and probably will not be available for human use for at least five years.

Current Research: New Medications

Between thirty and fifty new medications for treating various forms of heart disease are released every year. The majority of these are generic forms of existing trade-name drugs, or new medications in an already existing category of medications (see chapter 8). In a few areas, however, medical research may release some entirely new drugs during the next few years.

Monoclonal Anti-Platelet Antibodies

One of the risks of angioplasty is that the procedure may cause damage to the inside of the coronary artery, resulting in a blood clot that obstructs the artery and causes a heart attack. About 30 percent of people who undergo angioplasty are at high risk of developing this complication. Several methods are currently used to prevent the formation of blood clots following angioplasty in high-risk patients.

One of the more novel techniques uses antibodies, the proteins that the immune system makes to bind to an invading bacteria or virus. Monoclonal antibodies are antibody molecules made in a laboratory to attach to one specific substance. The FDA has recently approved (for limited use in high-risk angioplasty patients) a monoclonal antibody that binds to platelets, the small particles in the bloodstream that start blood clot formation.

When injected, the monoclonal antibody binds to platelets and helps prevent them from forming clots. An initial clinical trial with more than 2,000 high-risk coronary angioplasty patients indicated that use of this medication reduced the incidence of heart attacks and emergency coronary surgery following angioplasty.

The drug is not without risk, however. Use of the drug was associated with a significant increase in the incidence and severity of bleeding, which could result in major complications. For this reason its use is reserved for those patients at the highest risk of developing clots. The product's manufacturer has agreed to conduct further investigations into ways of reducing the risk of bleeding complications. In the meantime, its use is limited to very high-risk angioplasty patients.

Other Anti-Clotting Medications

While anti-platelet antibodies may be useful to treat high-risk patients for a short time, many heart patients can benefit from long-term use of medications that reduce the tendency to form blood clots. Currently the only medications widely used for this purpose are aspirin, which modestly interferes with platelets, and anticoagulants such as coumadin, which are difficult for doctors and patients to regulate. At this time, almost a dozen anti-clotting medications with several very different mechanisms of action are being studied in animals, and a few are entering human trials.

Several of these medications act specifically on the lining of damaged blood vessels. These medications might effectively prevent blood clots from forming in the coronary arteries, while avoiding the bruising and bleeding tendency that accompanies the current anticoagulants. Other medications act either on the platelets or on the clotting chemicals in the blood, but could have advantages over currently available medications. One or two of these medications could be available within the next few years.

New Evidence Concerning HMG-CoA Reductase Inhibitors

The HMG-CoA reductase inhibitors (see chapter 8) have been widely used to lower serum cholesterol and low-density lipoprotein levels, reducing the risk of continued atherosclerosis. Recent studies have demonstrated clearly that at least one drug in this class, pravastatin (Pravachol) does in fact lower the mortality rate of people who take it following a heart attack.

While these results do not immediately change the way doctors will treat patients after heart attacks, other research has begun on more specific ways to use these drugs in persons with coronary artery disease. It is possible that these studies will show that these drugs could benefit even people who have normal cholesterol levels. They also may (or may not) be more appropriate for coronary artery disease patients than are the other types of cholesterol-lowering drugs.

Reteplase

Reteplase is a new thrombolytic drug used to treat persons within the first two hours after a heart attack. It is very similar in action to the other drugs in this class (see chapter 2) and has not been shown to be more effective than they are. It has the unique advantage of being administered in a simple two-injection method, rather than by a complex constant infusion. It is thought that the simpler method of administration will allow this drug to be administered more rapidly to heart attack patients than the other drugs in this class. It may also reduce the chance of underdose or overdose in this situation. Reteplase is now being released for general use.

Circadian Timed-Release Medications

The circadian rhythm is the twenty-four-hour internal clock of the body. It has long been known that many of the body's hormones and other functions vary depending on the time of day (this is most obvious if you've ever suffered jet lag). Many hormones that affect blood pressure and the heart show variations according to the circadian rhythm.

Some new drug delivery systems are designed to release the drug in time with the body's circadian rhythm. They are taken once a day at bedtime. They then release medication at different rates during the next twenty-four hours, allowing the dose to reflect the hormonal state of the body. Theoretically, this should allow better control of blood pressure and other functions that are known to vary according to the circadian rhythm.

Currently, a circadian release version of verapamil is available for the treatment of high blood pressure and angina. While the drug has been documented to be useful, it has not been shown for certain that it is superior to other forms of verapamil. Several other types of antihypertension medications are also being developed as circadian release medicines.

Current Research: New Tests for Heart Disease

Ultrafast CT Scan

Computed tomography (CT) scans have long been used to give overall cross-sectional pictures of the heart and chest. Because the movement of the beating heart is too fast for the machine to capture an image, pictures of the heart's structures are blurry and out of focus. For this reason they are of limited usefulness in visualizing the heart valves or other structures.

New "ultrafast" CT scans can take an image so quickly that the movements of normal heartbeats do not interfere with their pictures. They can be used to visualize the valves and even the larger parts of the coronary arteries. Because CT scans require no catheters or other equipment to be inserted into the body, they are safer than some types of cardiac tests. They cannot show the amount of blockage in a coronary artery, however, only whether some blockage is present. Because of this limitation, ultrafast CT scans will probably be used only as a screening test. They will not replace angiography or other types of cardiac tests.

Positron Emission Tomography

Positron emission tomography (PET) scans can provide detailed, three-dimensional views of the internal organs (similar to those of a CT scan).

They also provide information about the biochemical makeup of the various tissues of the body. Because of this ability, several current studies are determining how PET scans can be used to diagnose heart disease. Although many of the things PET scans can demonstrate are also visualized by other studies, there is some indication that PET scans may provide invaluable information for treating patients, especially those who have both coronary artery disease and congestive heart failure.

In people with both these diseases, many different tests, including angiography, nuclear scans, and ultrasound, show that some segments of the heart muscle fail to contract. Some of these areas are scar tissue caused by old heart attacks, but others are parts of the heart muscle that are in "hibernation." Hibernation of heart muscle occurs when the muscle has enough oxygen supply to survive, but not enough to allow it to contract. The muscle stops contracting in order to stay alive. If blood supply to such areas is restored by CABG or angioplasty, then the muscle will begin contracting again, decreasing the degree of congestive heart failure.

Until recently, physicians made an educated guess of whether there was "hibernating" heart muscle after weighing the information from other tests. PET scans, however, can tell exactly how much muscle remains alive but hibernating. This allows physicians to decide whether a procedure to restore blood flow is likely to benefit a person in congestive heart failure. The PET scan technology is already widely available, although it is not yet commonly used for this purpose.

Should You Participate in Clinical Trials?

New technology is available in clinical trials well before it is available to the general public. If you are treated at a large medical center or medical school, you may be offered the opportunity to participate in a clinical trial of a new technology or new medication. Even if you are not seen in such a center, your doctor may discuss referring you to one if you have a condition that is appropriate for such a trial.

Participating in clinical trials carries some advantages and also some risks. Obviously, you may be given access to a new medication or technology sooner than you would otherwise, but remember there is no guarantee that the new treatment will work or be more effective than the treatment you would get otherwise. Often, however, you will receive free medication, tests, and other care while you participate in the trial, and these costs savings might be a significant benefit for you. Many studies also provide much more in-depth monitoring and continuing care than would otherwise be available to you.

On the other hand, you will be required to take certain medications or treatments exactly as they are prescribed. Every study has strict guidelines on patient compliance. If you don't follow the guidelines exactly, you will be removed from the study. You will also undergo more tests and be seen by the doctors performing the study more frequently than you would if you were simply being treated for your condition. If the study center is located far from your home, this could be inconvenient. Most studies also have carefully designed criteria of medical conditions, age, and other factors that determine who can participate. Even if you want to be part of the study, you may not qualify.

Finally, most medication studies and some treatment studies are "double blind." This means that half the patients receive the study medication, while the other half receive a standard treatment or a placebo. If you participate in such a study, neither you nor the doctors involved will know which medication you are receiving. Other studies are "crossover" studies. This means that you will receive the treatment part of the time and a standard medication (or placebo) part of the time. Again, neither you nor the doctors will know which medication you are receiving during either phase of the study.

All studies, however, have criteria to "unblind" the medication in the event of any endangerment of the patient. For example, if your condition deteriorates during the study, the doctor can "unblind" you and determine which medication you are receiving. If you have gotten worse while using the study medication it will be stopped immediately. If you have gotten worse when the study medication was removed, the doctor usually will be allowed to restart it even though it is not approved for general use.

In summary, there are clear reasons for some people to participate in clinical trials: No other treatment may be available, the cost savings may be important, or the patients may have a deep desire to help advance what medical science can do for their condition. For other people, participating in a medical study may have no clear benefit. Even though studies are carefully designed to minimize the risks involved, such people may be better off staying with accepted medical treatment.

CHOLESTEROL AND FAT CONTENT OF FOODS

Food	Serving Size	Total Fat (gm)	Saturated Fat (gm)	Cholesterol (mg)
Beverages				
Alcoholic beverages (including beer and wine)	6 oz.	0	0	0
Coffee				
Black, unsweetened	6 oz.	0	0	0
Cafe Francais	6 oz.	3.4	2.9	0
Cafe Vienna	6 oz.	2.4	2.1	0
Irish Mocha Mint	6 oz.	2.6	2.2	0
Suisse Mocha	6 oz.	2.8	2.4	0
Juices				
Apple	8 oz.	0.3	0	0
Cranberry	8 oz.	0.1	0	0
Grape	8 oz.	0.2	0.1	0
Orange	8 oz.	0.1	0	0
Prune	8 oz.	0.1	0	0
Tomato	8 oz.	0.2	0	0

Food	Serving Size	Total Fat (gm)	Saturated Fat (gm)	Cholesterol (mg)
Apple	8 oz.	0.3	0	0
Cranberry	8 oz.	0.1	0	0
Grape	8 oz.	0.2	0.1	0
Orange	8 oz.	0.1	0	0
Prune	8 oz.	0.1	0	0
Tomato	8 oz.	0.2	0	0
Soda, carbonated drinks	12 oz.	0	0	0
Tea	6 oz.	0	0	0

Breads and Noodles

Food	Serving Size	Total Fat (gm)	Saturated Fat (gm)	Cholesterol (mg)
Bagel	1	1.4	0.2	0
Biscuit	1	3.3	1.2	0
Bread, French	1 slice	1.0	0.2	0
Bread, raisin	1 slice	1.0	0.3	0
Bread, wheat	1 slice	1.1	0.3	0
Bread, white	1 slice	0.9	0.2	0
Cornbread	1 slice	4.0	1.5	34
Crescent roll	1	5.0	2.7	6
English muffin	1	1.1	0.2	0
Kaiser roll	1	8.1	1.3	4
Macaroni	1 oz.	0.4	0	0
Muffin, bran	1	5.1	1.8	26
Muffin, blueberry	1	4.3	1.3	25
Noodles, egg	1 cup	2.4	0.8	50
Noodles, ramen	1 cup	6.8	1.5	0
Pancake	1	3.2	1.2	27
Spaghetti noodles	1 cup	0.7	0.1	0
Stuffing from mix	½ cup	12.2	3.0	1
Waffle, frozen	1	3.2	1.0	24

Candy

Food	Serving Size	Total Fat (gm)	Saturated Fat (gm)	Cholesterol (mg)
Almond Joy	1	7.8	3.6	1
Butterscotch hard candy	3 pieces	7.0	6.0	0
Caramels	3 pieces	2.9	1.3	8
Chocolate	1 oz.	9.0	5.0	5

Food	Serving Size	Total Fat (gm)	Saturated Fat (gm)	Cholesterol (mg)
Chocolate chips	¼ cup	12.2	6.3	1
Chocolate-covered almonds	1 oz.	12.1	4.2	3
Chocolate-covered peanuts	1 oz.	9.0	2.6	1
Hard candy (except butterscotch)	1 oz	0.3	0	0
Jelly beans	1 oz.	0	0	0
Marshmallows	1 oz.	0	0	0
Milky Way	1	9.0	4.7	6
Mr. Goodbar	1	15.0	7.8	7
Nestle Crunch	1	8.0	5.0	6
Reese's Peanut Butter Cup	1	10.7	6.0	5
Snickers	1	13.0	4.4	3

Cereals

Food	Serving Size	Total Fat (gm)	Saturated Fat (gm)	Cholesterol (mg)
All-Bran	1 oz.	0.5	0	0
Alpha Bits	1 oz.	0.6	0.1	0
Bran Flakes	1 oz.	0.5	0.1	0
Cap'n Crunch	1 oz.	2.6	1.7	0
Cheerios	1 oz.	1.8	0.3	0
Cornflakes	1 oz.	0.1	0	0
Cream of Wheat	1 oz.	0.4	0.1	0
Frosted Mini-Wheat	1 oz.	0.3	0	0
Granola	1 oz.	4.9	3.3	0
Grits	1 oz.	0.5	0	0
Kix	1 oz.	0.7	0.2	0
Oatmeal	1 oz.	1.7	0.3	0
Product 19	1 oz.	0.2	0	0
Raisin Bran	1 oz.	0.5	0.1	0
Rice Krispies	1 oz.	0.2	0	0
Shredded Wheat	1 oz.	0.3	0.1	0
Special K	1 oz.	0.1	0	0
Total	1 oz.	0.6	0.1	0
Wheaties	1 oz.	0.5	0.1	0

Food	Serving Size	Total Fat (gm)	Saturated Fat (gm)	Cholesterol (mg)
Chips				
Cheese Balls, baked	1 oz.	6.0	1.5	1
Cheese Puffs	1 oz.	10.6	2.6	1
Corn chips (Fritos)	1 oz.	9.7	1.6	0
Pork rinds	1 oz.	9.3	3.7	24
Potato chips, plain	1 oz.	9.8	2.6	0
Potato chips, sour cream	1 oz.	9.5	2.6	1
Pretzels	1 oz.	1.0	0.5	0
Pringles, low-fat	1 oz.	7.0	2.0	0
Tortilla chips	1 oz.	7.0	1.1	0
Dairy Products				
Butter	1 pat	4.0	2.5	11
Cheese, American	1 oz.	8.9	5.6	27
Cheese, American low-fat	1 oz.	2.0	1.3	10
Cheese, cheddar	1 oz.	9.4	6.0	30
Cheese, cottage	1 oz.	5.1	3.2	17
Cheese, cottage low-fat	1 oz.	1.2	0.7	5
Cheese, cream	1 oz.	9.9	6.2	31
Cheese, mozzarella	1 oz.	7.0	4.4	25
Cheese, Swiss	1 oz.	7.8	5.0	26
Cream	1 oz.	2.9	1.8	10
Cream, artificial creamer	1 pack	0.7	0.7	0
Cream, sour	1 tbsp.	2.5	1.6	5
Cream, whipped	1 tbsp.	5.6	3.5	21
Cream, artificial whipped topping	1 tbsp.	0.7	0.4	2
Ice Cream	1 cup	23.7	14.7	88
Ice Cream, low-fat	1 cup	14.0	8.9	59
Ice Milk	1 cup	5.6	3.5	18
Milk, whole	1 cup	8.2	5.1	33
Milk, 2%	1 cup	4.7	2.9	18
Milk, skim	1 cup	0.4	0.3	4
Yogurt	1 cup	7.4	4.8	29

Food	Serving Size	Total Fat (gm)	Saturated Fat (gm)	Cholesterol (mg)
Cheesecake	1 slice	14.3	8.9	30
Chocolate cake with icing	1 slice	10.8	5.5	26
Chocolate chip cookie	1	2.3	0.9	4
Custard	½ cup	7.3	3.5	154
Danish pastry	1	4.9	1.8	9
Doughnut	1	5.8	2.7	23
Doughnut, glazed	1	9.2	4.5	15
Eclair	1	15.4	7.3	195
Fig bar	1	1.0	0.4	6
Gelatin	1	0	0	0
Oatmeal cookie	1	3.2	1.1	13
Pecan pie	1	23	5.6	30
Pound cake	1	8.8	304	51
Sugar cookie	1	3.4	1.4	6

Eggs

Food	Serving Size	Total Fat (gm)	Saturated Fat (gm)	Cholesterol (mg)
Egg (1)	1	5.6	1.7	210
Egg white	1	0	0	0
EggBeater's egg substitute	1	0	0	0

Fruit

Food	Serving Size	Total Fat (gm)	Saturated Fat (gm)	Cholesterol (mg)
Apple	1	0.5	0.1	0
Banana	1	0.6	0.2	0
Cantaloupe	½	0.4	0	0
Coconut, fresh	¼ cup	15.1	13.4	0
Figs	3	0.2	0	0
Grapefruit	½	0.1	0	0
Orange	1	0.1	0	0
Peach	1	0.1	0	0
Pear	1	0.7	0	0
Plum	1	0.4	0	0
Raisins		0.5	0.2	0
Strawberries		0.5	0	0

Food	Serving Size	Total Fat (gm)	Saturated Fat (gm)	Cholesterol (mg)
Margarine and Cooking Oils				
Fats				
Beef	1 tbsp.	12.8	6.4	14
Chicken or turkey	1 tbsp.	12.8	3.8	11
Lard	1 tbsp.	12.8	5.0	12
Margarine	1 tbsp.	3.8	0.7	0
Oils				
Canola (rapeseed)	1 tbsp.	13.6	0.9	0
Coconut	1 tbsp.	13.6	8.1	0
Cottonseed	1 tbsp.	13.6	3.5	0
Olive	1 tbsp.	13.6	1.8	0
Palm	1 tbsp.	13.6	8.8	0
Peanut	1 tbsp.	13.6	2.3	0
Safflower	1 tbsp.	13.6	1.2	0
Sesame	1 tbsp.	13.6	1.9	0
Sunflower	1 tbsp.	13.6	1.4	0
Shortening	1 tbsp.	12.8	3.2	0
Meats (assumes lean cuts) and Fish				
Beef				
Brisket	3 oz.	13.5	5.3	77
Chuck roast	3 oz.	13	5.3	90
Flank steak	3 oz.	13.2	5.6	60
Ground beef	3 oz.	15.7	6.2	74
Liver	3 oz.	4.2	1.6	331
Porterhouse steak	3 oz.	18.0	7.5	70
Ribs	3 oz.	15.4	6.6	79
Round steak	3 oz.	12.6	4.8	81
Veal cutlet	3 oz.	5.7	2.5	84
Bologna	3 oz.	8.0	3.0	16
Fish and Shellfish				
Catfish	3 oz.	3.6	0.8	49
Clams	3 oz.	1.7	0.2	57

Food	Serving Size	Total Fat (gm)	Saturated Fat (gm)	Cholesterol (mg)
Cod	3 oz.	0.7	0.1	47
Crab	3 oz.	1.5	0.2	85
Fishsticks (breaded)	3 oz.	12.2	3.1	112
Halibut	3 oz.	2.5	0.4	35
Herring	3 oz.	9.9	2.2	65
Lobster	3 oz.	0.5	0.1	61
Orange roughy	3 oz.	7.0	0.1	20
Oysters	3 oz.	2.1	0.5	47
Salmon	3 oz.	5.3	1.4	41
Scallops	3 oz.	0.5	0.1	28
Shrimp (boiled)	3 oz.	0.9	0.2	166
Snapper	3 oz.	1.5	0.3	40
Tuna (light, in oil)	3 oz.	7.0	1.3	15
Tuna (light, in water)	3 oz.	0.4	0.1	15
Frankfurter	1	13.2	4.8	45
Frankfurter, turkey	1	8.0	2.2	48
Lamb	3 oz.	6.9	2.3	71
Pork				
Bacon	3 oz.	9.4	3.3	16
Canadian bacon	3 oz.	3.9	1.3	27
Ham	3 oz.	9.4	3.2	80
Loin	3 oz.	11.8	4.1	77
Shoulder	3 oz.	12.7	4.4	82
Poultry (Note: At least double these values if skin is left on. Increase total fat 1 gm if fried.)				
Chicken breast, skinless	1	3.1	0.9	73
Chicken drumstick, skinless	1	2.5	0.7	71
Chicken liver	3 oz.	3.8	1.3	442
Chicken thigh, skinless	1	5.4	1.5	49
Turkey breast, skinless	1	0.8	0.3	73
Turkey drumstick, skinless	1	8.5	2.8	170
Salami	3 oz.	3.9	0.9	23

Food	Serving Size	Total Fat (gm)	Saturated Fat (gm)	Cholesterol (mg)
Sausage				
Italian	3 oz.	7.3	2.6	11
Kielbasa	3 oz.	7.7	2.8	19
Polish	3 oz.	8.1	2.9	20
Pork (breakfast)	3 oz.	8.4	2.9	22
Snacks				
Cracker Jacks	1 oz.	1.0	0.1	0
Crackers				
Cheese	2	4.9	1.2	4
Graham	2	1.5	0.6	3
Ritz	2	2.9	0.8	5
Saltine	2	0.6	0.2	2
Wheat Thins	2	1.4	0.4	2
Granola bar	1	5.0	4.3	0
Nuts				
Almonds	1 oz.	9.5	0.9	0
Cashews	1 oz.	13.2	2.6	0
Peanuts	1 oz.	14.0	1.9	0
Pecans	1 oz.	19.2	1.5	0
Pistachios	1 oz.	15.0	1.9	0
Olives				
Black	2	4.0	0.5	0
Green	2	1.6	0.2	0
Pickles	2	0.2	0	0
Popcorn	1 oz.	0.7	0.3	0
Sunflower seeds	1 oz.	14.1	1.5	0
Vegetables				
Artichoke	1	0.2	0	0
Avocado	1	27	4.5	0
Barley	1 cup	0.5	0	0
Beets	1 cup	0.1	0	0

Food	Serving Size	Total Fat (gm)	Saturated Fat (gm)	Cholesterol (mg)
Carrots	1 cup	0.2	0	0
Cauliflower	1 cup	0.2	0	0
Celery	1 cup	0.1	0	0
Corn	1 cup	0.8	0.1	0
Green beans	1 cup	0.2	0	0
Mushrooms	1 cup	0.2	0	0
Onion	1 cup	0.1	0	0
Peas	1 cup	0.5	0.1	0
Potato	1 cup	0.1	0	0
Rice	1 cup	0.2	0	0
Sauerkraut	1 cup	0.2	0	0
Squash	1 cup	0.2	0	0
Sweet potato	1	0.5	0.1	0
Tomato	1	0.3	0	0
Beans				
BBQ with sauce	1 cup	4.0	1.5	1
Black-eyed peas	1 cup	0.4	0.2	0
Butter	1 cup	0.6	0.1	0
Garbanzo	1 cup	2.4	0.5	0
Kidney	1 cup	0.4	0.1	0
Lima	1 cup	0.7	0.2	0
Split peas	1 cup	0.3	0.1	0
White	1 cup	0.6	0.2	0

RESTAURANT AND PREPARED FOOD GUIDE

Food	Calories	Total Fat (gm)	Cholesterol (mg)
Canned and Bottled Foods			
Beef stew	145	4.0	47
Chili and beans	390	26.0	52
Clam chowder	163	6.6	22
Corned beef hash	184	12.5	35
Franks and beans	355	14.0	8
Salad dressings (per tablespoon)			
Blue cheese	77	8.0	3
French, low-calorie	22	0.9	1
Italian, low-calorie	16	1.5	1
Mayonnaise, regular	100	11.0	8
Thousand Island	76	7.8	2
Sauces and gravy (per cup)			
Barbecue sauce	188	4.5	0
Beef gravy	124	5.5	7

Food	Calories	Total Fat (gm)	Cholesterol (mg)
Mushroom sauce	70	0.9	1
Soy sauce	11	0	0
Teriyaki sauce	15	0	0
Soup (per cup)			
Beef broth	16	0.5	0
Chicken broth	39	1.4	1
Chicken noodle	53	1.2	7
Cream of chicken	233	14.7	20
Cream of mushroom	255	19.0	2
Minestrone	83	2.5	2
Tomato	86	1.9	0
Vegetable	80	1.9	0
Vegetable beef	79	1.9	5

Frozen Foods

Food	Calories	Total Fat (gm)	Cholesterol (mg)
Beef Enchiladas (El Charrito)	260	11.0	25
Beef pie (Banquet)	409	20.0	65
Chicken a la king (Banquet)	138	4.7	36
Chicken enchiladas (Healthy Choice)	270	4.0	25
Chicken fettuccine (Healthy Choice)	260	4.5	40
Chicken pie (Swanson)	780	44.0	80
Egg rolls (La Choy)	120	5.2	45
Lasagna (Stouffer's)	385	14.0	90
Rice and chicken (Stouffer's)	270	8.0	20
Pizza, cheese (Celeste)	320	12.8	32
Pizza, cheese (Tombstone)	380	19.0	50
Pizza, sausage (Celeste)	367	16.8	52
Swedish meatballs (Budget)	550	34.0	160

Restaurant Fast Food

Abby's

Food	Calories	Total Fat (gm)	Cholesterol (mg)
Roast beef sandwich	353	15.0	39
Chicken breast sandwich	592	27.0	57
Fries (small)	211	8.0	6

Food	Calories	Total Fat (gm)	Cholesterol (mg)
Burger King			
Whopper	628	36.0	90
Hamburger	275	12.0	37
Chicken Tenders	204	10.0	47
Fries (small)	227	13.0	14
Church's			
Chicken breast, fried	278	17.3	n/a
Chicken thigh, fried	306	21.6	n/a
Catfish, fried	201	12.0	n/a
Kentucky Fried Chicken			
Chicken breast, original	276	17.3	96
Chicken breast, extra-crispy	354	23.7	66
Chicken thigh, original	278	19.2	122
Chicken thigh, extra-crispy	371	26.3	121
Baked beans	105	1.2	0.4
Biscuit	269	13.6	0
McDonald's			
Big Mac	570	35.0	83
Egg McMuffin	340	16.0	5.9
Quarter Pounder	427	24.0	81
Fillet-O-Fish	435	26.0	47
Chicken McNuggets	323	20.0	62
Fries (small)	220	11.5	9
Pizza Hut			
Thin crust, cheese	450	15.0	n/a
Thick crust, cheese	560	14.0	n/a
Thin crust, Supreme	510	21.0	n/a
Taco Bell			
Beef burrito	466	21.0	n/a
Taco	186	34.0	n/a
Wendy's			
Big Classic	470	25.0	80
Chicken breast sandwich	340	13.0	60
Baked potato, w/sour cream	465	24.0	15
Chili	240	8.0	25
Frosty (small)	400	14.0	50

MEDICATION NAMES AND CLASSIFICATION BY TRADE NAME

Trade Name	Generic Name	Classification
Adalat	Nifedipine	Calcium Channel Blocker
Aldactone	Spironolactone	Potassium-Sparing Diuretic
Aldomet	Methyldopa	Antihypertensive
Altace	Ramipril	ACE Inhibitor
Apresoline	Hydralazine	Antihypertensive
Aquatensin	Methyclothiazide	Thiazide Diuretic
Blocadren	Timolol	Beta Blocker
Bumex	Bumetanide	Loop Diuretic
Calan	Verapamil	Calcium Channel Blocker
Capoten	Captopril	ACE Inhibitor
Cardene	Nicardipine	Calcium Channel Blocker
Cardilate	Erythrityl tetranitrate	Nitrate
Cardioquin	Quinidine	Antidysrhythmic
Cardizem	Diltiazem	Calcium Channel Blocker
Catapres	Clonidine	Antihypertensive
Cordarone	Amiodarone	Antidysrhythmic

Trade Name	Generic Name	Classification
Corgard	Nadolol	Beta Blocker
Crystodigin	Digitoxin	Inotrope
Dilantin	Phenytoin	Antidysrhythmic
Dilatrate	Isosorbide dinitrate	Nitrate
Diuril	Chlorothiazide	Thiazide Diuretic
Duraquin	Quinidine	Antidysrhythmic
DynaCirc	Isradipine	Calcium Channel Blocker
Dyrenium	Triamterene	Potassium-Sparing Diuretic
Edecrin	Ethacrynic Acid	Loop Diuretic
Enduron	Methyclothiazide	Thiazide Diuretic
Esidrix	Hydrochlorothiazide	Thiazide Diuretic
HydroDiuril	Hydrochlorothiazide	Thiazide Diuretic
Hygroton	Chlorthalidone	Thiazide Diuretic
Inderal	Propranolol	Beta Blocker
Isoptin	Verapamil	Calcium Channel Blocker
Isordil	Isosorbide dinitrate	Nitrate
Lanoxin	Digoxin	Inotrope
Lasix	Furosemide	Loop Diuretic
Loniten	Minoxidil	Antihypertensive
Lopressor	Metoprolol	Beta Blocker
Lotensin	Benazepril	ACE Inhibitor
Mexitil	Mexilitine	Antidysrhythmic
Midamor	Amiloride	Potassium-Sparing Diuretic
Minipress	Prazosin	Antihypertensive
Monopril	Fosinopril	ACE Inhibitor
Nitro-Bid	Nitroglycerine	Nitrate
Nitro-Disc	Nitroglycerine	Nitrate
Nitro-Dur	Nitroglycerine	Nitrate
Nitrogard	Nitroglycerine	Nitrate
Nitrol Ointment	Nitroglycerine	Nitrate
Nitrolingual	Nitroglycerine	Nitrate
Nitrostat	Nitroglycerine	Nitrate
Normodyne	Labetalol	Beta Blocker, Alpha Blocker

Trade Name	Generic Name	Classification
Norpace	Disopyramide	Antidysrhythmic
Oretic	Hydrochlorothiazide	Thiazide Diuretic
Peritrate	Pentaerythrityl tetranitrate	Nitrate
Plendil	Felodipine	Calcium Channel Blocker
Prinivil	Lisinopril	ACE Inhibitor
Procan	Procainamide	Antidysrhythmic
Procardia	Nifedipine	Calcium Channel Blocker
Pronestyl	Procainamide	Antidysrhythmic
Quinaglute	Quinidine	Antidysrhythmic
Quinalin	Quinidine	Antidysrhythmic
Quinidex	Quinidine	Antidysrhythmic
Rhythmol	Propafenone	Antidysrhythmic
Sectral	Acebutolol	Beta Blocker
Sorbitrate	Isosorbide dinitrate	Nitrate
Tambocor	Flecainide	Antidysrhythmic
Tenormin	Atenolol	Beta Blocker
Thalitone	Chlorthalidone	Thiazide Diuretic
Tonocard	Tocainide	Antidysrhythmic
Trandate	Labetalol	Beta Blocker, Alpha Blocker
Transderm-Nitro	Nitroglycerine	Nitrate
Tridil	Nitroglycerine	Nitrate
Vascor	Bepridil	Calcium Channel Blocker
Vasotec	Enalapril	ACE Inhibitor
Verelan	Verapamil	Calcium Channel Blocker
Visken	Pindolol	Beta Blocker
Wytensin	Guanabenz	Antihypertensive
Zaroxolyn	Metolazone	Thiazide Diuretic
Zestril	Lisinopril	ACE Inhibitor

MEDICATION NAMES AND CLASSIFICATION BY GENERIC NAME

Generic Name	Trade Name	Classification
Acebutolol	Sectral	Beta Blocker
Amiloride	Midamor	Potassium-Sparing Diuretic
Atenolol	Tenormin	Beta Blocker
Benazepril	Lotensin	ACE Inhibitor
Bepridil	Vascor	Calcium Channel Blocker
Bumetanide	Bumex	Loop Diuretic
Captopril	Capoten	ACE Inhibitor
Chlorothiazide	Diuril	Thiazide Diuretic
Chlorthalidone	Hygroton Thalitone	Thiazide Diuretic
Clonidine	Catapres	Antihypertensive
Digitoxin	Crystodigin	Inotrope
Digoxin	Lanoxin	Inotrope
Diltiazem	Cardizem	Calcium Channel Blocker
Enalapril	Vasotec	ACE Inhibitor
Erythrityl tetranitrate	Cardilate	Nitrate

Generic Name	Trade Name	Classification
Ethacrynic Acid	Edecrin	Loop Diuretic
Felodipine	Plendil	Calcium Channel Blocker
Fosinopril	Monopril	ACE Inhibitor
Furosemide	Lasix	Loop Diuretic
Guanabenz	Wytensin	Antihypertensive
Hydralazine	Apresoline	Antihypertensive
Hydrochlorothiazide	Esidrix HydroDiuril Oretic	Thiazide Diuretic
Isradipine	DynaCirc	Calcium Channel Blocker
Isosorbide dinitrate	Isordil Sorbitrate Dilatrate	Nitrate
Labetalol	Normodyne Trandate	Beta Blocker, Alpha Blocker
Lisinopril	Zestril Prinivil	ACE Inhibitor
Methyclothiazide	Aquatensin Enduron	Thiazide Diuretic
Methyldopa	Aldomet	Antihypertensive
Metolazone	Zaroxolyn	Thiazide Diuretic
Metoprolol	Lopressor	Beta Blocker
Minoxidil	Loniten	Antihypertensive
Nadolol	Corgard	Beta Blocker
Nicardipine	Cardene	Calcium Channel Blocker
Nifedipine	Procardia Adalat	Calcium Channel Blocker
Nitroglycerine	Nitrostat Nitrogard Nitrolingual Nitrol ointment Nitro-Bid Nitro-Dur Nitro-Disc Transderm-Nitro Tridil	Nitrate

Generic Name	Trade Name	Classification
Pentaerythrityl tetranitrate	Peritrate	Nitrate
Pindolol	Visken	Beta Blocker
Prazosin	Minipress	Antihypertensive
Propranolol	Inderal	Beta Blocker
Ramipril	Altace	ACE Inhibitor
Spironolactone	Aldactone	Potassium-Sparing Diuretic
Timolol	Blocadren	Beta Blocker
Triamterene	Dyrenium	Potassium-Sparing Diuretic
Verapamil	Calan Isoptin Verelan	Calcium Channel Blocker

STOP-SMOKING RESOURCES

Most of these sources will send information about various stop-smoking plans and will refer you to local support groups and services at no charge. A few of the most complete national resources are identified with an asterisk (*). When a site has an Internet address, this is included. A separate section identifies Internet-only resources.

Some for-profit commercial resources are included that supply specific or hard-to-locate services. Their inclusion here does not constitute a recommendation by the author. Rather it is the author's intention to include any possible service that might help any reader quit smoking.

General Sources

American Academy of
  Otolaryngology, Head, and
  Neck Surgery
One Prince Street
Alexandria, VA 22314
1-800-393-6733
(Pamphlets on quitting.)

American Cancer Society*
4 West 35th Street
New York, NY 10001
1-800-227-2345
www.cancer.org/
("Fresh-Start" program and "I Quit
Kit" by mail. The ACS also sponsors
four-week quit-smoking group sessions in many areas of the U.S.)

American Health Association
7320 Greenville Avenue
Dallas, TX 75231
(214) 822-9380
(Pamphlets: "Calling It Quits,"
"Guidelines for Weight Control.")

American Lung Association*
1740 Broadway
New York, NY 10019-4374
(212) 315-8700
(Pamphlets: "Freedom from
Smoking," "Stop Smoking—
Stay Trim," and others.)

American Tobacco Information
    Network (ATIN)
1-800-432-2772
(Smoking cessation programs
in Arizona.)

Black Health Education Council
1721 2nd Street, Suite 101
Sacramento, CA 95814
(916) 556-3344 (tel.)
(916) 446-0427 (fax)

Center for Substance Abuse
    Treatment (CSAT)
    (a division of the U.S. Public
    Health Service)
Office of the Director
(301) 443-5700 (tel.)
(301) 443-8751 (fax)
http://treatment.org/csat.html
(attempts to support local
smoking cessation groups.)

Massachusetts Tobacco Control
    Program
Massachusetts Department of
    Public Health
250 Washington Street, 4th Floor
Boston, MA 02108-4619
Massachusetts Smoker's Quitline
1-800-TRYTOSTOP
(Free help for smokers in this area)

Nicotine Anonymous*
Dept. A, P.O. Box 591777
San Francisco, CA 94159-1777
(415) 327-6734
(415) 750-0328 (national hotline)
http://www.nicotine-anonymous.org

Office on Smoking and Health
    (OSH)
National Center for Chronic Disease
    Prevention and Health
    Promotion (NCCDPHP)
Centers for Disease Control and
    Prevention (CDC)
4770 Buford Highway, N.E.
Atlanta, GA 30341-3724
Mail Stop K-50
(770) 488-5705
1-800-CDC-1311 (voice mail, fax
    information)
http://www.cdc.gov/nccdphp/osh/
    tobacco.html

Commercial Services

American Healthways
1739 E. Broadway Road, Suite 309
Tempe, AZ
spyndr@ix.netcom.com
(Herbal stop-smoking aids.)

DynaGen, Inc.
99 Erie Street
Cambridge, MA 02139
(617) 491-2527 (tel.)
(617) 354-3902 (fax)
(Saliva nicotine test strips.)

LungCheck Inc.
8255 E. Raintree Drive
Scottsdale, AZ 85260
1-800-456-5864
http://www.LungCheck.com/
(Provides tests to check for pre-cancerous cells in the sputum.)

Nicotine Dependence Center
Mayo Clinic
200 First Street
Rochester, MN 55905
(Program for "hard-core" smokers claims 54% success, costs about $3,000, and involves an 8 day inpatient treatment including counseling and nicotine replacement therapy.)

SmokEnders National Offices
3708 Diablo Boulevard
Lafayette, CA 94549
1-800-828-4357
www.smokenders.com
(Comercial program, costs about $125 for a "quit kit". 81% of people who complete the 7 week program quit smoking.)

SmokerNot
2599 E. Main Street, Suite 217
Columbus, OH 43209
(614) 236-4644

International Resources

All Africa Conference on Tobacco
 or Health (AACToH)
P.O. Box 29356
Sunnyside, 0132, South Africa
Contact: Dr. Derek Yach
 0927-12-341-4313 (tel.)
 0927-12-341-0510 (fax)
Dr. Yussuf Saloojee
 (011) 640-2058 (tel.)
 (011) 720-6177 (fax)

Asian Consultancy on Tobacco
 Control
Riftswood, 9th milestone, DD 229
Lot 147, Clearwater Bay Road
Sai Kung, Kowloon, Hong Kong

BC Doctors' Stop-Smoking Program
1665 W. Broadway
Vancouver, BC V6J 5A4
(504) 736-4566
http://www.cma.ca/e-pubs/smoking/
 index.html

Canadian Cancer Society
116 Albert Street
Ottawa, Ontario, K1P 5V5, Canada
(613) 567-3050 (tel.)
(613) 567-5695 (fax)
http: //www.ccsh.ca/ncth

European Consultancy on Tobacco
 Control
c/o Dr. H. P. Adriaanse, Associate
 Professor,
Department of Health Education,
University of Limburg
P.O. Box 616
6200 MD Maastricht, Netherlands
31(0) 43-882224/882406 (tel.)
31(0) 43-671032 (fax)
adriaanse@gvo.rulimburg

International Agency on Tobacco
 and Health/Action on Smoking
 or Health (ASH)
109 Gloucester Place
London, W1H 3PH, England
44-071-935-3519 (tel.)
44-071-935-3463 (fax)

National Clearinghouse on Tobacco
 and Health (Canada)
1000-170 Laurier Avenue West
Ottawa, Ontario, K1P 5V5, Canada
(613) 567-3050 (tel.)
(613) 567-5695 (fax)
http://www.ccsh.ca/ncth

Sources on the Internet

Netwellness
University of Cincinnati Medical
    Center
http://www.netwellness.org
(Broad range of online help, also
provides local referrals in the
Cincinnati area.)

National Institutes of Health
http://search.info.nih.gov
(Large searchable database about
the effects of smoking, some information about quitting.)

QuitNet
http://www.quitnet.org/
(Large number of links to stop-
smoking programs. A lot of for-
profit companies connect here.)

Tobacco Bulletin Board System*
http://www.tobacco.org/
(Huge number of links to both
commercial and not-for-profit stop-
smoking groups, as well as a large
number of online documents about
stop-smoking aids.)

RESOURCES FOR PERSONS WITH CARDIAC DISEASE

Books, pamphlets, and journal articles take at least several months to be published and distributed. The most up-to-date information can often be found on Internet sites. Whenever possible, Internet addresses have been included to allow you to get the newest information. Most public libraries have Internet access computers available to the general public and will be happy to show you how to access these sites.

General Information About Heart Disease

American Heart Association
7320 Greenville Avenue
Dallas, TX 75231
(214) 822-9380
1-800-527-6941
www.amhrt.org
(Web site describes many different materials they offer, but does not allow you to download the material directly. Please order this information through the mail or by phone.)

American Heart Association (DC)
1250 Connecticut Avenue, N.W.
Washington, DC 20036
(202) 822-9380

American Medical Association
   Division of Cardiology
535 North Dearborn Street
Chicago, IL 60610
(312) 645-4419

National Center for Health
   Statistics
6525 Belcrest Road, Room 1064
Hyattsville, MD 20782
(301) 436-8500

Information About New Treatment Options and Clinical Trials

Cardiovascular Institute of the South
www.cardio.com
(Site gives a wealth of information
in clearly organized, easy to understand articles, most of which can
be downloaded.)

Cholesterol, Genetics, and Heart
   Disease Institute
http://www.heartdisease.org/
(This site is provided for physicians,
but it goes to great pains to make
its information quite readable to
non-physicians.)

Clinical Trials Center
http://www.centerwatch.com//
   LISTING.HTML
(Keeps a current list of ongoing
clinical trials that are actively
recruiting patients. Although it
has a subsection for heart disease,
you may have to scroll through a
long list of studies to find any
pertinent information for your
condition.)

The Congenital Heart Disease
   Resource Page
http://www.csun.edu/~hcmth011/
   heart
(Superb privately maintained page
links you to information on most
types of congenital heart disease.)

Foundation for Making Informed
   Medical Decisions
http://www.dartmouth.edu/dms/cec/
   fimdm/
(Excellent page that really tries to
show the facts for several heart
conditions that have different
treatment options.)

Heart Information Network
http://www.heartinfo.org
(A fair amount of general information.)

Medical Education Discussion
   Forum for Risk Reduction in
   Coronary Artery Disease
Internet Medical Education, Inc.
http://www.med-edu.com/

MedSeek
http://medseek.com/
(Physician and hospital referral
service that lists 280,000 physicians
by specialty. Recommends some
outstanding doctors on the basis of
other doctors' referrals. Useful if
you are having trouble finding the
right specialist.)

National Heart, Lung, and Blood
   Institute
P.O. Box 30105
Bethesda, MD 20824-0105
(301) 951-3260
(301) 951-3269
http://www.nhlbi.nih.gov/nhlbi.html
(Large searchable database about
heart disease treatments and prevention.)

National Institute of Health
Bethesda, MD 20894
(301) 496-6308
http://search.info.nih.gov
(Large searchable database about
heart disease, as well as information
about clinical trials and current
research.)

National Organization for Rare
   Disorders, Inc.
P.O. Box 8923
New Fairfield, CT 06812-8923
1-800-999-6673
http://www.stepstn.com/nord/
   org_sum/1587.html
(Provides information to people
about rare and unusual disorders.
Excellent site for information about
unusual congenital heart defects
and rare forms of heart disease.)

Netwellness
University of Cincinnati Medical
   Center
http://www.netwellness.org
(Broad range of online information,
also provides local referrals in the
Cincinnati area.)

University of California,
   San Francisco Medical School
Galen Search Engine
http://www.library.ucsf.edu/search.
   html
(Allows you to search for information by topic. The site can provide a
lot of information but is confusing
to learn and can be difficult to use.)

WellnessWeb
http://wellweb.com
(This site was founded by patients
who discovered how difficult it is to
become well enough informed to
communicate with their doctors.
Provides excellent information for
heart patients. Does have a few
commercially sponsored links, but
even these are useful.)

Heart Patient Recovery and Support Groups

Children's Heart Society
www.childrensheart.org
(Information and support for
congenital heart defects.)

HeartLink
18 Briar Walk, Fishponds
Bristol, BS16 4JJ, England
http://www.ibmpcug.co.uk/
44-117-904-6224 (tel.)
44-117-904-6223 (fax)
Freephone UK 0500-676670
(Good information source on
recovery. Also provides support
for patients and families via
online discussion groups and in
person in Great Britain.)

Mended Hearts
National Office
Dallas, TX 75231
(214) 706-1442
Also can be reached through the
American Heart Association:
1-800-AHA-USA1
www.mendedhearts.org.
(Volunteers who visit patients
at more than 400 hospitals. Has
chapters in many major cities.)

Minnesota Heart Health Program
Stadium Gate 20
611 Beacon Street U.M.
Minneapolis, MN 55455
(612) 624-1818

Support Group Communications
http://www.support-group.com/
    links/heart_disease/index.html
(Site listing a number of local and
regional support groups for heart
patients, may help you find a local
support group. Also has links to
some on-line support groups.)

INDEX